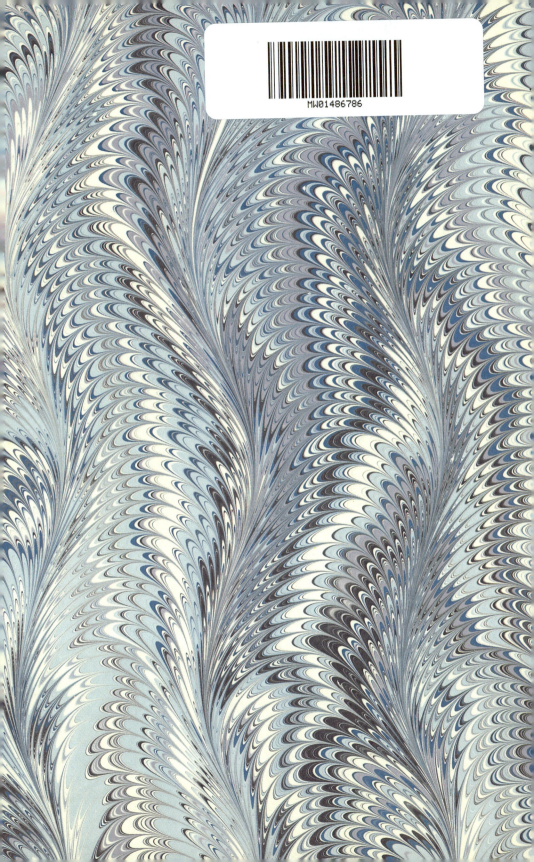

REMEMBER YOUR RUBBERS!

COLLECTIBLE CONDOM CONTAINERS

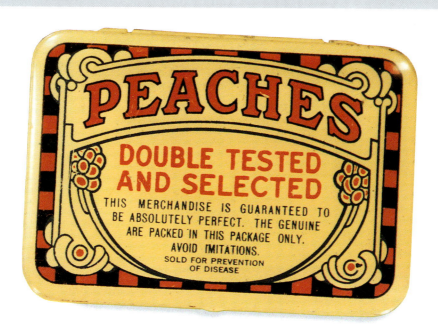

G.K. Elliott - George Goehring - Dennis O'Brien

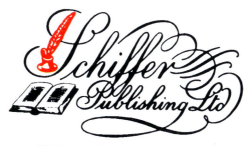

Schiffer Publishing Ltd

4880 Lower Valley Road, Atglen, PA 19310

Book design by Blair Loughrey

ISBN: 0-7643-0414-3
Printed in China
1 2 3 4

Published by Schiffer Publishing Ltd.
4880 Lower Valley Road
Atglen, PA 19310
Phone: (610) 593-1777; Fax: (610) 593-2002
E-mail: Schifferbk@aol.com
Please write for a free catalog.
This book may be purchased from the publisher.
Please include $3.95 for shipping.
Please try your bookstore first.

We are interested in hearing from authors
with book ideas on related subjects.

If you have any questions about rubber containers
please feel free to call Dennis and George at (410) 889-
3964, or G.K. Elliot at (303) 797-8069.

CONTENTS

FOREWORD

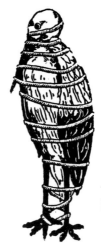

The Stork
Ensnared

Antique rubber containers are rapidly increasing in value, attracting much attention from collectors as well as organizations interested in promoting safe sex. In short they're not just hot. They're positively scorching!

Notwithstanding the current craze, these little fellows have always been desirable and very elusive. The main reason for their scarcity is that people didn't keep them around to store things in, as they did other early advertising containers. We hear stories of rare tobacco or coffee cans filled with everything from sewing items to nuts and bolts, discovered in some basement, attic, or drawer. Not so when it comes to rubber tins! Not only were they too small for storing things, but people were much too embarrassed to keep them around and, despite their beautiful graphics, hastily discarded them after use.

So if they aren't found in basements, attics and drawers, where are they found? This is one of the really fun, interesting facts about rubber containers—*where* they're found! For instance, many have been discovered in old fishing tackle boxes. What were those boys really up to when they told their wives they were going off on a weekend fishing trip? Rubber tins have also been found in the back seats of old Chevies with fuzzy dice on the mirrors. The "Rough Rider" pictured in this book was found in a barn, probably used in a hurry and tossed in the hayloft where it was left to rust. The tin is "rough," indeed, but it is the only example to have ever surfaced.

Our favorite "location" was discovered by a vintage clothing dealer who found a rubber tin in a World War II sailor's hat! It was hidden inside in a little hand-sewn pocket, made just to hold a ready stash for a chance onshore rendezvous. The dealer said she wouldn't have noticed it had she not accidentally felt a little bulge in the hatband. That tin was the "Radium Nutex" pictured in this book!

CHAPTER 1
CAOUTCHOUC

In the words of the great tin can authority, Nosmo King: "They're rubbers, damn it! Condoms are for wimps!" We owe the word "rubber" to Joseph "The Gasman" Priestley, famous mad scientist, who was the first to "rub out" pencil marks with a "rubber" (eraser) in 1770. Before that, the stuff was called caoutchouc (cowchock) a South American Indian word meaning weeping wood. The strange spelling is due to a short involvement with a Frenchman. It wasn't until the 1930s that people started to use the words "rubber" for tires and balls, and "latex" for gloves and rubbers.

The Mayans were the first people to extract latex and use it to make balls, about one thousand years ago. Then Columbus, on his second voyage to the "New World," found the natives of Haiti playing with caoutchouc balls. He snagged a few as presents for the court of Isabella. Later, in 1735, French explorers published the first scientific reports on caoutchouc samples collected in Amazonia, and in 1803 the first caoutchouc factory opened near Paris.

When it came to clothing, cloth was first treated with a waterproof solution of turpentine and rubber in 1791. It stayed flexible but the stink never faded. The first popular rainwear for tradesmen, the Macintosh, made in 1823, was made of a sandwich of canvas held together by a solution of latex and naphtha. In 1826 Macintosh and Hancock formed a partnership to develop caoutchouc goods and its processes.

In the winter of 1843, Charles Goodyear invented what was to be one of the great economic milestones of the rubber industry—vulcanization. This produced a durable product that could be used for cigar cases, portable darkrooms, rubber baby buggy bumpers, capotes anglaises, French letters, and male safes.

The first rubbers (condoms) were made from sheets of crepe rubber derived by spreading out a sheet of Macintosh's naphtha solution, which was dried, cut to size and cemented together with the same solution. Later, these seamed goods were

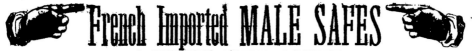
Ad for rubbers 1865. 7-1/8" x 4-1/2". *Courtesy of James C. Frasca.*

replaced by cement rubbers, a seamless product made by dipping a glass or ceramic form in cement, letting it dry, then vulcanizing it by exposure to sulfur dioxide. Since a few people had a reaction to naphtha or sulfur, the rubber was dipped in kerosene as a neutralizer. To prevent a rash from contact with the kerosene, the rubber was finally dipped in an acid bath…thus replacing the rash with blisters. All this chemical prevention did nothing for the taste.

The alternatives were either an animal membrane or, the favorite of the United States Army through both World Wars, the famous chemical prophylactic that replaced blisters with screaming and a rash. It wasn't until the nineteenth century that the new water-cured liquid latex process was invented. For the most part, this hypoallergenic process was a true boon to man (and woman) kind. More improvements occurred in the 1960s and 1970s, including colored latex (cool), flavored latex (icky), and, in the 1980s, the amazing glow in the dark latex (sold as a novelty only).

Novelty Rubbers

Right from the start, jokers have inserted rubbers into candy and cookies. In 1863 G.S. Haskins Inc., 36 Beekman Street, New York City, offered "lascivious candy and lovers sweetmeats, each piece featuring a superior condom." Nut trees, like filberts and walnuts, can be induced to form a shell over a rubber. Naturally, you

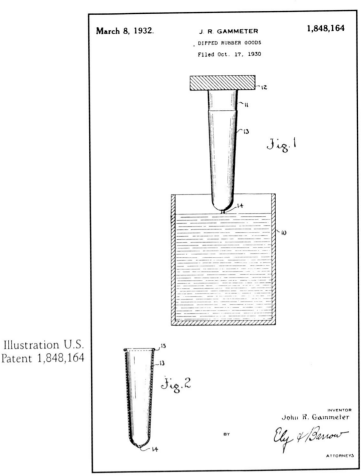

Illustration U.S.
Patent 1,848,164

can get damn near anything in a golf ball. Another popular trick is to disguise a rubber as something more innocuous. The list includes cigarettes and cigarette packs (popular in Japan and Korea), folding matchbooks (complete with faux matches & striker), faux lipstick (Queen-Tex), and key chains. Rubbers have also appeared as earrings and inside greeting cards. The high-tech award goes to "Frederick's of Hollywood" for the electronic pressure sensitive musical condom, "The Wedding Surprise."

Distribution

Rubbers have been found in drugstores, machines, newsstands, shoeshine parlors, pool halls and "the bastion of male chauvinism," barber shops. During World War II, The United States Army maintained posts to issue free rubbers (often in front of brothels). Rubber salesmen were referred to as "Pencil Men." Orders were placed as "a gross of Trojan pencils" to avoid any embarrassment from overheard phone conversations.

Above:
Order form 1956. H. Hanson Sales. 8-1/2" x 11.

Left:
Illustration U.S. Patent 5,163,447

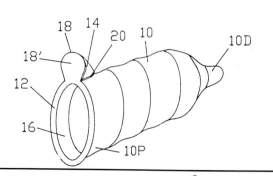

CHAPTER 2
PACKAGING

Paper Packaging

Interestingly enough, both the oldest and newest rubber packages are envelopes. India rubbers, latex rubbers and animal membrane prophylactics are found in envelopes. Most hold one dozen rubbers lying flat, though a few can be found with one quarter dozen. "Genuine Liquid Latex" rubbers came packaged with four (rolled) to an envelope and wrapped in cellophane. Rarer are envelopes with a single rubber in the package. The largest variety of rubbers came in machine dispenser packs. The earliest came from the 1930s and they are still made. Machine packs can hold one to three rubbers. In the 1940s the packs became cellophane wrapped. During World War II, at least three manufacturers made paper boxes as part of the war effort to conserve metal. Some say "war package" on the back. These boxes came both hinged and "shell & slide," like matchboxes. All metal rectangular containers were shipped in paper boxes in unit counts of 4, 12 and 48.

By the 1950s rubbers evolved to sealed packets of cellophane, metal foil, and plastic. The first pre-lubricated rubbers, like "Dean's Redi-Wet Peacocks," came in foil. Most machine packets have a foil packet inside. Foil packets leave the famous tell-tail wallet ring, the "mark of honor" for many baby boomers.

Metal Boxes.

Three types of prophylactics came in metal containers: India rubber, liquid latex, and chemical. No animal membrane prophylactics have been found in a metal container. The oldest containers were round and made of aluminum. The aluminum containers were all embossed with no color printing and none list manufacturers. Most are thought to have been made between World War I and the mid-1930s. Of all the aluminum containers, "Three Merry Widows" offered the most variations in design.

The next developments were both round and square tins exhibiting color lithography. The rectangle (hinged) box was introduced later. All round containers are friction fit. Of the three types rectanglular containers are the most numerous. The earliest known hinged rectangles appeared in the late 1920s. All metal containers held three rolled rubbers, and the packaging often refers to the contents as "one quarter dozen." Tins were discontinued in the late 1950s.

UNITED STATES PATENT OFFICE

2,347,719

CONTAINER

Edward O. Then, Newark, N. J., assignor to American Can Company, New York, N. Y., a corporation of New Jersey

Application July 8, 1939, Serial No. 283,465

2 Claims.   (Cl. 220—36)

The present invention relates to a two-part hinged tablet box or container and has particular reference to an improved construction which provides for easy opening of the box.

An object of the invention is the provision of a two-part hinged tablet box or the like wherein the cover part is retained on the body part by a floating pintle hinge and wherein pivot projections formed on the cover part rest on the upper edge of the body part adjacent the hinge and thus provide fulcrum points on which the cover may be easily rocked by pinching the rear edge of the box so that the latter may be readily snapped open with one hand.

Numerous other objects and advantages of the invention will be apparent as it is better understood from the following description, which, taken in connection with the accompanying drawing, discloses a preferred embodiment thereof.

Referring to the drawing:

Figure 1 is a perspective view of a box embodying the instant invention, the view showing the box being snapped open, the view showing the outline of a portion of a hand in such operation of pinching the box.

Fig. 2 is a rear elevation of the box shown in Fig. 1,

Figs. 3 and 4 are enlarged sections taken substantially along the line 3—3 in Fig. 2 and showing the cover of the box in different positions, and

Fig. 5 is a section taken substantially along the line 5—5 in Fig. 3.

As a preferred embodiment of the invention the drawing illustrates a tablet box which includes a sheet metal body member 11 and a sheet metal cover member 12 which is retained on the body member by a hinge 13. The body member is preferably of a one piece die drawn construction which comprises a rectangular shaped flat bottom wall section 15 having a surrounding upright and continuous side wall which includes a front wall section 16, a rear wall section 17, and a pair of connecting side wall sections 18. At the corners these sections are curved or rounded as indicated by the numeral 19.

The construction of the cover member 12 is similar to the construction of the body member 11 and preferably includes a semi-flattened, dome shaped top wall section 21 which is surrounded by a continuous depending and integral flange 22. The flange includes a front wall section 23, a rear wall section 24, and a pair of connecting side wall sections 25. The corners of these wall sections are rounded as at 26 to fit the body member.

At the rear of the box the cover member 12 and the body member 11 are hinged together in a floating pintle hinge. Such a hinge includes a pintle 31 which is tightly retained in a long hinge lug 32 formed in the rear flange wall section of the cover 12. The ends of the pintle extend beyond the ends of the lug 32 and are engaged in a pair of outwardly projecting hinge lugs 33 formed in the rear wall section 17 of the body member.

The body member hinge lugs 33 are vertically elongated in order to allow the pintle free vertical movement therein so that the hinge will be of a floating character. With this hinge construction the cover may be readily hinged back out of the way to gain access to the interior of the box.

When the cover member 12 is in closed position on the body member it preferably rests on the front edge of body wall section 16 and is locked against inadvertent opening. This locking feature is effected by a pair of small interlocking bosses 35, 36 which are pressed outwardly from the front wall sections 16 and 23 of the body member 11 and the cover member 12 respectively.

Provision is made for readily opening the box by pinching the rear edges of the cover and the body members together. For this purpose there is provided a small integrally struck indentation or inwardly extending projection 41 in the cover member 12 adjacent the juncture between its top wall 21 and each side wall 25 thereof. There are thus two of these projections, one on each side of the cover, and they are spaced equally forward from the hinge 13. When the cover is in closed position these projections rest on the upper edge at the rear of the side wall sections 18 of the body member. The projections 41 could be formed in the body side wall sections 18 if desired and thus have them engage against the edge of the cover member with the same operating effect.

Hence when the rear edge of the box is pinched, the hinge pintle 31 moves down in the elongated body lugs 33 and this action rocks the cover member 12 about its fulcrum or pivot projections 41. With this rocking movement the outer catch boss 36 in the front wall section 23 of the cover member snaps out of locking engagement with the inner catch box 35 of the front wall section 16 of the body member 11. At the same time the pintle 31 seats in its lugs 33 with the result that the front edge of the released cover is moved up and away from the body member and into an initial or partially opened position. From this initial position it is an easy matter to complete

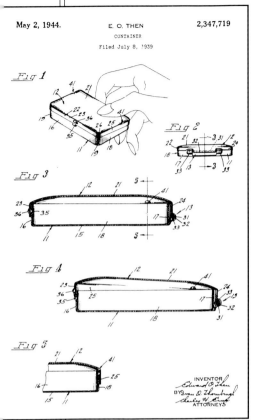

Illustration U.S.
Patent 2,347,719

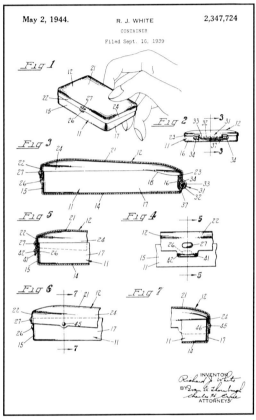

Illustration U.S.
Patent 2,347,724

Number 41

After years of mind numbing, dusty patent file "hide-and-seek," a treasure has been found: U.S. Patent 2,347,719 from July of 1939. On line 91 through line 101 it reads: "(41) Provision is made for readily opening the box by pinching the rear edges of the cover and the body members together" etc.

Much to our disappointment this cool device has no name! Henceforth it shall be known as "Number 41." Great expectations were held that this discovery might be of use for "dating" tin cans—romance is where you find it—but this device was in use long before any patent was filed.

CHAPTER 3
PAPER AND TIN CONTAINERS

Note: Due to the age of tins and to the photographic and printing process, colors may not reproduce to complete accuracy.

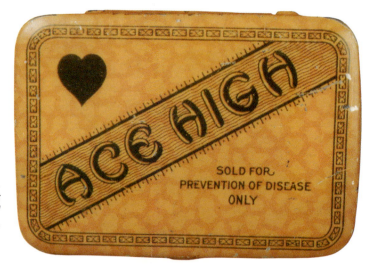

Ace High. Manufacturer unknown. 2-5/8" x 1-3/4". Rare.

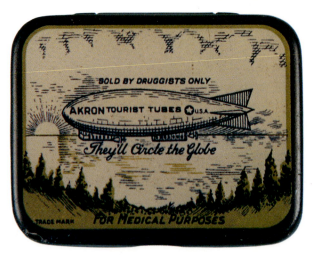

Akron Tourist Tubes (green mountains). Akron Rubber Supply Company. 2-1/8" x 1-5/8". Rare. A fitting start for a "Tour de Rubbers." A flying phallus out to "Circle the Globe." This rare tin came in the two color variations shown here.

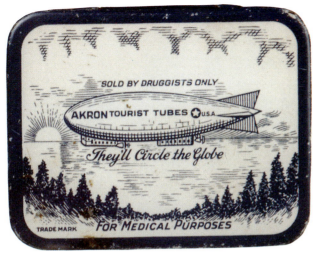

Akron Tourist Tubes (blue). Akron Rubber Supply Company. 2-1/8" x 1-5/8". Rare.

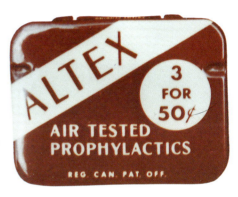

Altex (# 41) Western Rubber Company, Canada. 2-1/8" x 1-5/8". *Courtesy of Wm. Morford Auctions.* $650.

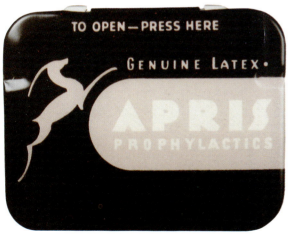

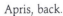

Apris, back.

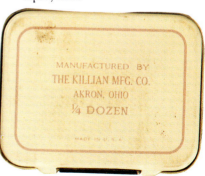

Apris (# 41), front. Killian Manufacturing Company. 2-1/8" x 1-5/8". $125.00

APRIS

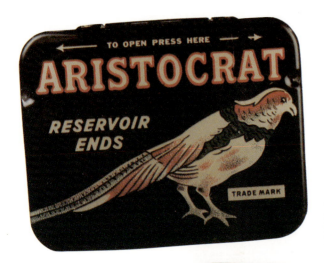

Aristocrat (# 41).
Midwest Drug
Company. 2-1/8" x
1-5/8". $450.00.

Aristocrat,
back.

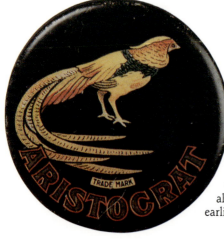

Aristocrat. 1-5/8" round.
Rare. No manufacturer is
listed but since the
rectangular Aristocrat came
from the Midwest Drug
Company, we assume they
also produced this beautiful
earlier version.

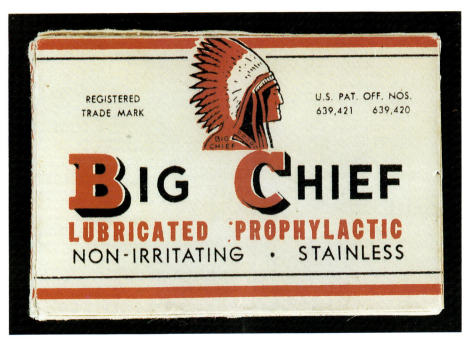

Big Chief. Contains one foil packet. H. L. Blake Company, Inc. 2-5/8" x 1-3/4". $20.00

Big Chief foil packet.

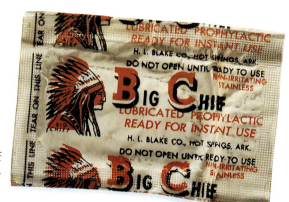

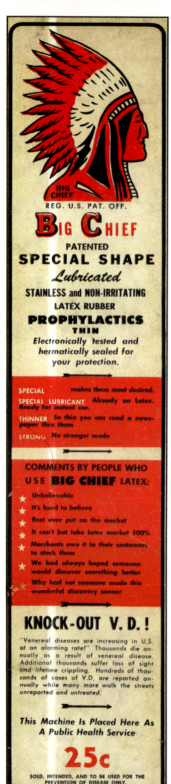

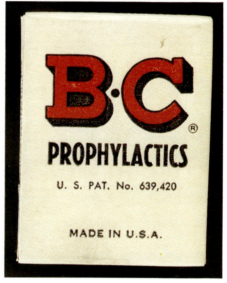

B.C. (paper). H. L. Blake Company, Inc. 2-1/8" x 1-5/8". $5.00

Big Chief. Decal for machine. 15-1/2" x 3-1/4".

16

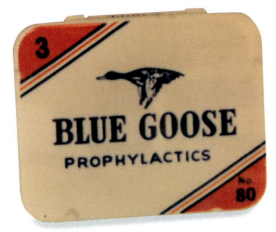

Blue Goose. Schaeffer Products. 2-1/4" x 1-3/4". *Courtesy of Wm. Morford Auctions.* Rare. Notice the resemblance to the hood ornaments of 1920s Ford automobiles.

Blue Goose, (# 41), reservoir ends. Schaeffer Products. 2-1/4" x 1-3/4". Rare.

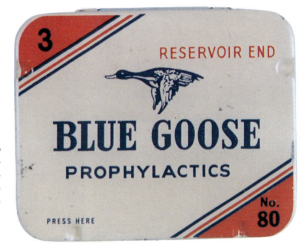

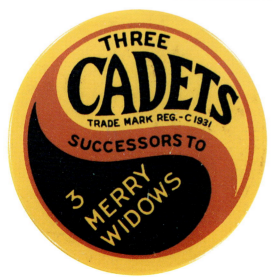

Cadets, yellow. Julius Schmid, Inc. 1-5/8" round. $200.00..

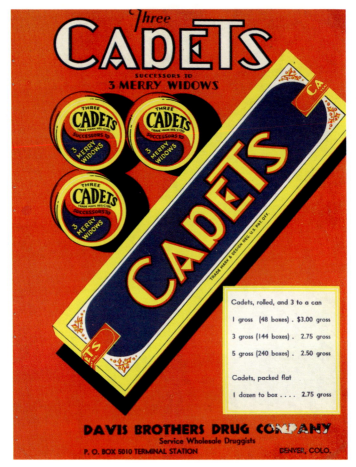

Cadets ad, 1930, front.

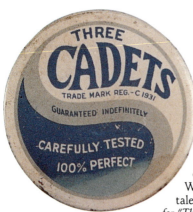

Cadets, blue. Julius Schmid, Inc. 1-5/8" round. Rare. "Cadets." U.S. Copyright files show the first use of this name as April-1934. Copyright number 371,561 was granted in 1938. The round blue tin is the hardest to find. Though we have seen many examples of the rectangle in 9 or better condition none have had the contents. In Denver, Colorado, before World War II, a "Cadet" was a person that recruited talent for brothels. (*See "Aluminum Containers" for "Three Merry Widows."*)

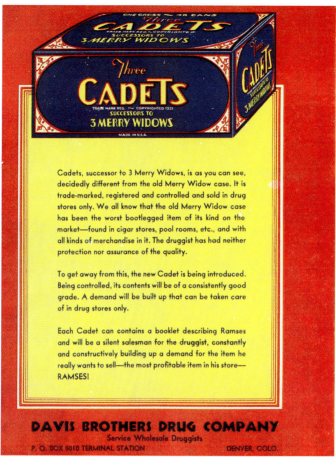

Cadets ad, 1930, back.

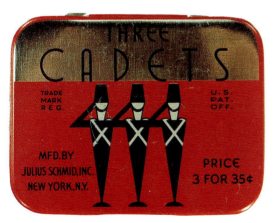

Cadets (front). Julius Schmid, Inc.
2-1/8" x 1-5/8". $125.00

Cadets, back.

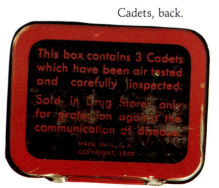

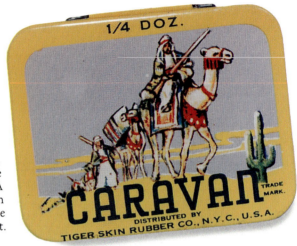

Caravan, yellow (front). Tiger Skin Rubber Company. 2-1/8" x 1-5/8". $170.00. Good use of artistic license. A Bedouin caravan passes through the Sonora Desert.

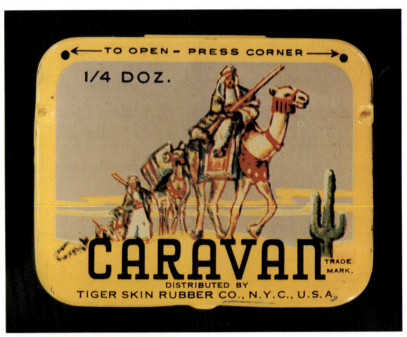

Caravan, (# 41), yellow, (front). Tiger Skin Rubber Company. 2-1/8" x 1-5/8".

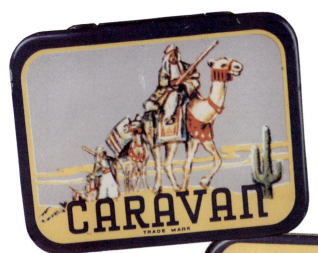

Caravan, (blue border). Tiger Skin Rubber Company. 2-1/8" x 1-5/8". Rare.

Caravan, back.

CARAVANS'

ARE MADE FROM STRONG, THIN LATEX RUBBER AND HAVE BEEN 100% BLOWN TESTED. FULLY INSPECTED FOR YOUR PROTECTION. ASK FOR CARAVANS BY NAME AT YOUR DRUGGIST. ACCEPT NO SUBSTITUTE. SOLD EXCLUSIVELY IN DRUG STORES AND FOR THE PREVENTION OF DISEASE ONLY.

DISTRIBUTED BY

TIGER SKIN RUBBER CO.

NEW YORK CITY, U. S. A.

MADE IN U.S.A.

A.C.CO.50AM

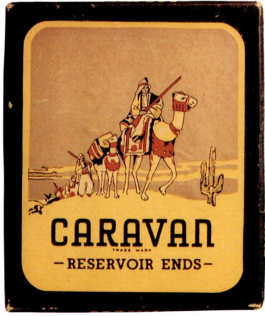

Caravan, (paper), one gross. Tiger Skin Rubber Company. $30.00

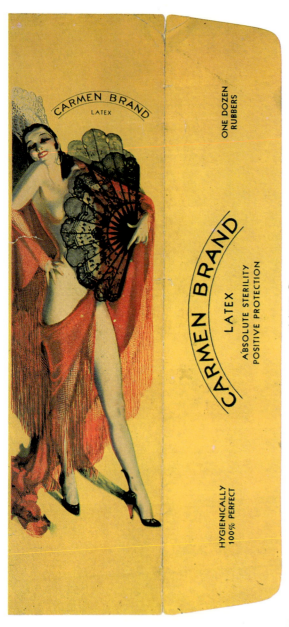

Carmen Brand
(paper), One Dozen.
Manufacturer
unknown. $30.00.

Carmen. Manufacturer
unknown. 1-5/8" round.
$450.00. This beauty is said to
be the work of pin-up artist Rolf
Armstrong. (see "Safway Brand").

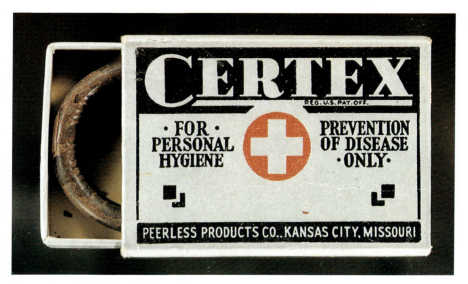

Certex (paper). Peerless Products Company.
2" x 1-3/8" shell & slide. $25.00.

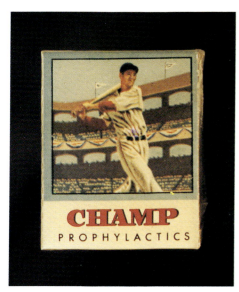

Champ (paper), baseball.
National Hygienic Products
Corporation. 2" x 1-5/8".
$125.00. This set of "sports"
is the most sought after of
the machine packs and can
be found in two versions
with or without zip codes.

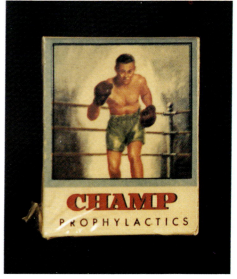

Champ (paper), boxing.
National Hygienic
Products Corporation.
2" x 1-5/8". $125.00.

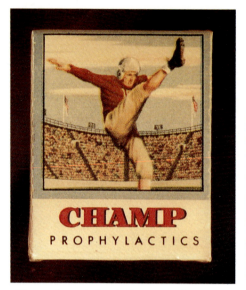

Champ (paper), football. National
Hygienic Products Corporation.
2" x 1-5/8". $125.00.

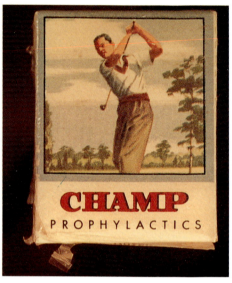

Champ (paper), golf. National
Hygienic Products Corporation.
2" x 1-5/8". $125.00.

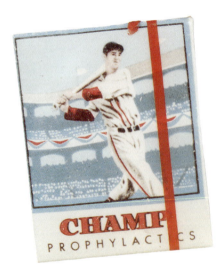

Champ (cardboard), baseball.
One dozen. National Hygienic
Products Corporation. 2-3/8" x
2-1/4" x 3/4". $200.00.

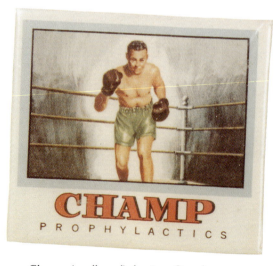

Champ (cardboard), boxing. One dozen.
National Hygienic Products Corporation.
2-3/8" x 2-1/4" x 3/4". $200.00.

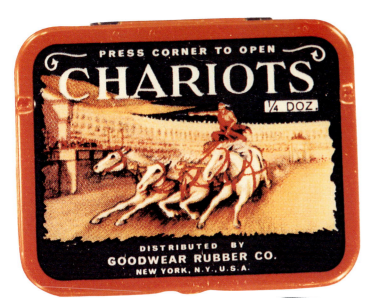

Chariots (# 41) (front). Goodwear Rubber Company. 2-1/8" x 1-5/8". $200.00. Ben-Hur whipping-on three white chargers, round the corner, at the circus-circus. Just sets spurs to the mind. Hi-Ho Goodwear!

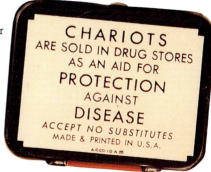

Chariots, back.

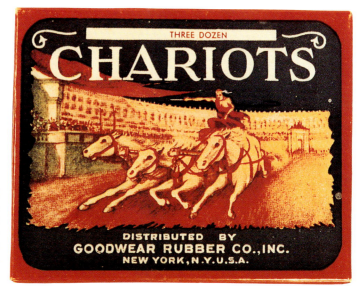

Chariots (paper) Three Dozen. Goodwear Rubber Company. 4-7/16" x 3-7/16". $20.00.

CHARIOTS

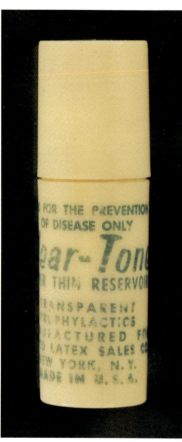

Cleartone (plastic). Allied Latex
Sales Company. 2-1/8" x 5/8"
round. $20.00.

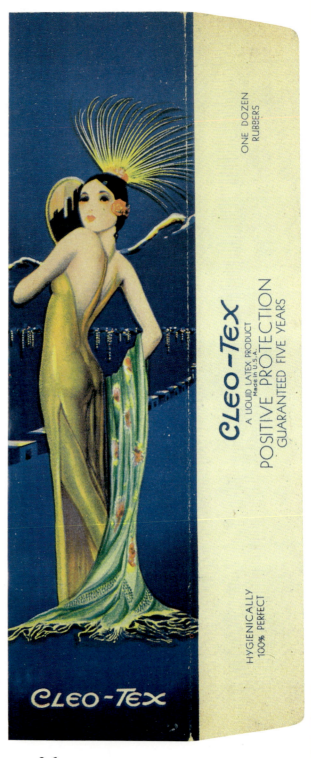

Cleo-Tex (paper),
One Dozen.
Manufacturer
unknown. $30.00

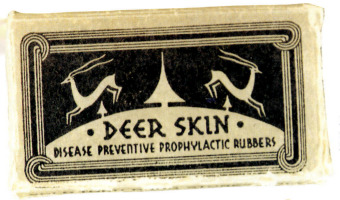

Deer Skin. Manufacturer unknown. 2" x 1-1/16". $5.00.

Deer Skin (paper), one dozen. Manufacturer unknown. 2-1/4" x 2". $5.00.

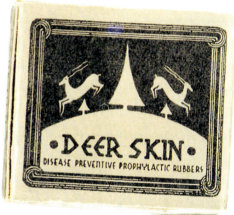

De-Luxe Blue-Ribbon. American Hygienic Company. 2-1/8" x 1-5/8". Rare. A very rare puppy.

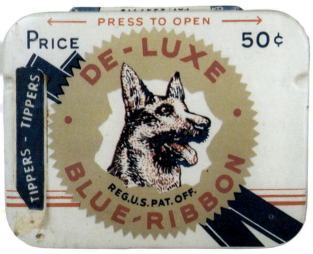

DE—LUXE

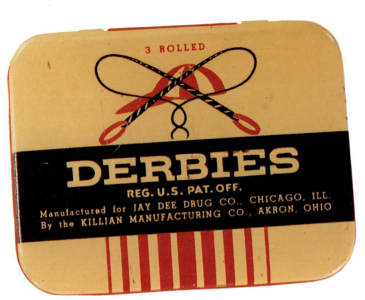

Derbies, front. Killian
Manufacturing Company.
2-1/8" x 1-5/8". $250.00

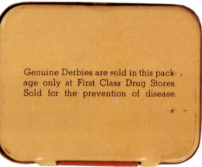

Genuine Derbies are sold in this package only at First Class Drug Stores.
Sold for the prevention of disease.

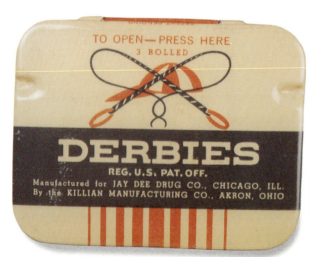

Derbies (# 41). Killian
Manufacturing Company.
2-1/8" x 1-5/8". $250.00.

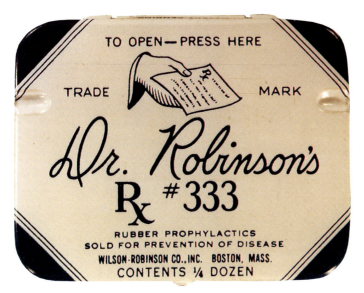

Dr. Robinson's RX #333 (# 41), front. Wilson-Robinson Company, Inc. 2-1/8" x 1-5/8"". $75.00.

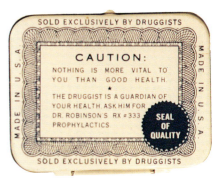

Dr. Robinson's RX #333, back.

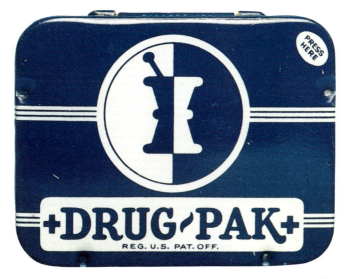

Drug-Pak (# 41). Nutex Sales Company. 2-1/8" x 1-5/8". $350.00

Duble-Tip, front. Department Sales
Company. 2-1/8" x 1-5/8". $750.00.

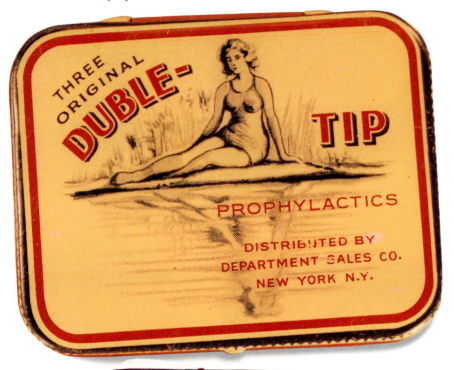

THREE ORIGINAL
DUBLE-
TIP

PROPHYLACTICS

DISTRIBUTED BY
DEPARTMENT SALES CO.
NEW YORK N.Y.

SOLD THROUGH DRUG
STORES ONLY.
—
INSIST ON GENUINE
DUBLE-TIP.

Made in U. S. A.

Duble-Tip,
back.

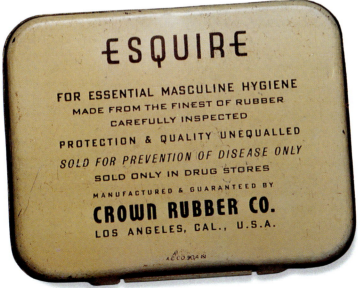

Esquire, front. Crown Rubber Company. 2-1/8" x 1-5/8". Rare. No relation to *Esquire Magazine*; its first issue was in the fall of 1933.

ESQUIRE

FOR ESSENTIAL MASCULINE HYGIENE
MADE FROM THE FINEST OF RUBBER
CAREFULLY INSPECTED

PROTECTION & QUALITY UNEQUALLED
SOLD FOR PREVENTION OF DISEASE ONLY
SOLD ONLY IN DRUG STORES
MANUFACTURED & GUARANTEED BY

CROWN RUBBER CO.
LOS ANGELES, CAL., U.S.A.

Esquire, back.

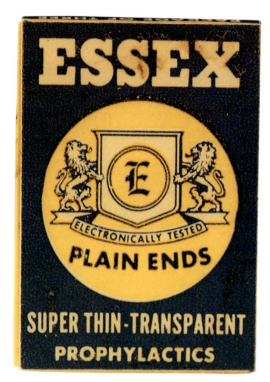

Essex (paper). Circle
Rubber Corporation.
2-1/8" x 1-1/2".
$5.00

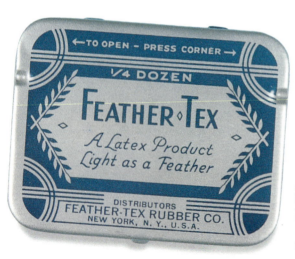

Feather-Tex (#41).
Feather-Tex Rubber
Company. 2-1/8" x
1-5/8". Rare.
Courtesy Bob Falck

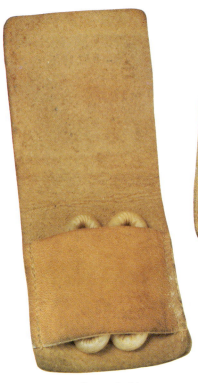

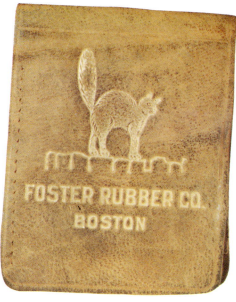

Foster Rubber Company (leather), front. *Courtesy of Steve & Donna Howard.* 2" x 2-3/4". Rare.

Foster Rubber Company, interior.

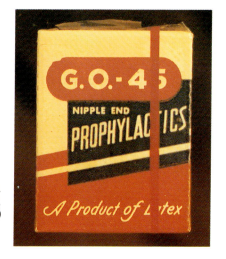

G.O. - 45 (paper).
2-1/8" x 1-1/2".
$5.00

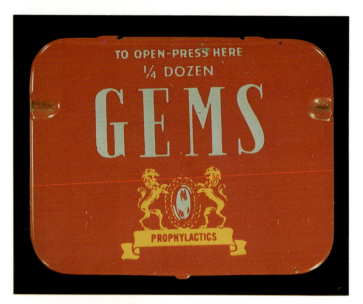

Above:
Gems (# 41), front. Allied Latex Sales Division. 2-1/8" x 1-5/8". $200.00

Left:
Gems, back.

Gems (paper). Allied Latex Sales Division. 2-1/8" x 1-1/2". $5.00.

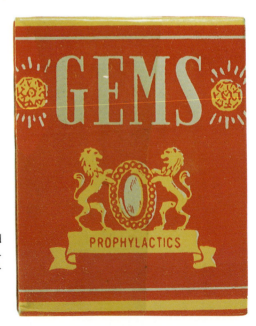

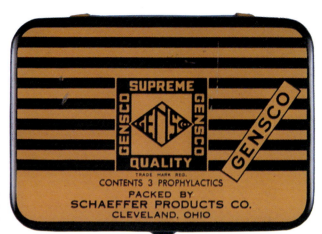

Gensco. Schaeffer Products Company. 2-1/2" x 1-3/4". $300.00.

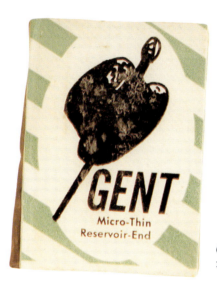

Gent (paper). 2-1/8" x 1-1/2". $5.00

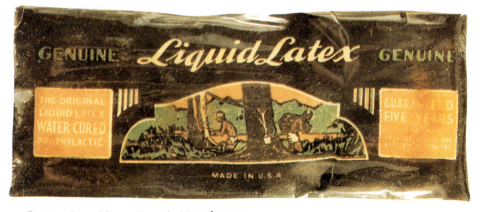

Genuine Liquid Latex (paper). Manufacturer unknown. 4-1/4" x 1-3/4". $10.00.

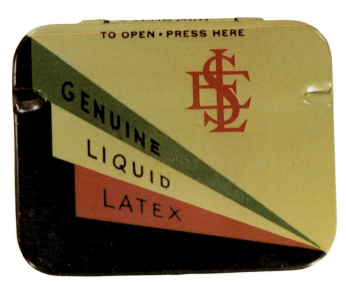

Genuine Liquid
Latex, L.E.S. (# 41).
L.E. Shunk Latex
Products, Inc. 2-1/8"
x 1-5/8". $100.00.

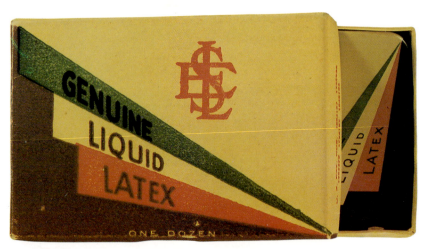

Genuine Liquid Latex, L.E.S. (paper), one dozen.
Held four tins. 3-1/2" x 3-3/8". $10.00.

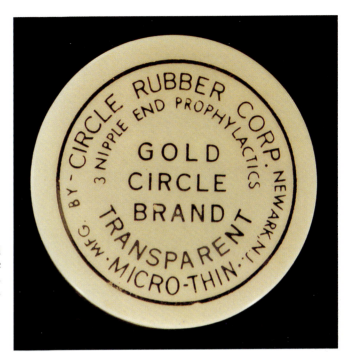

Gold Circle Brand
(plastic). Circle
Rubber Corporation.
1-3/4" round. $10.00.

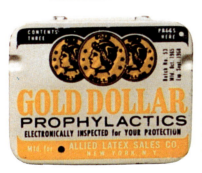

Gold Dollar (# 41). Allied
Latex Sales Company.
Courtesy of Michael Kain.
2-1/8" x 1-5/8". Rare.

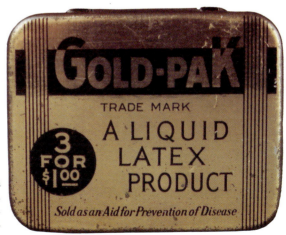

Gold-Pak. Crown
Rubber Company.
2-1/8" x 1-5/8".
$300.00.

37

GOLD–PAK

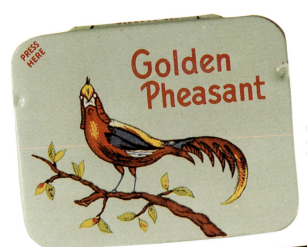

Golden Pheasant (# 41), front. W.H. Reed & Company, Inc. 2-1/8" x 1-5/8". $100.00

Golden Pheasant, back.

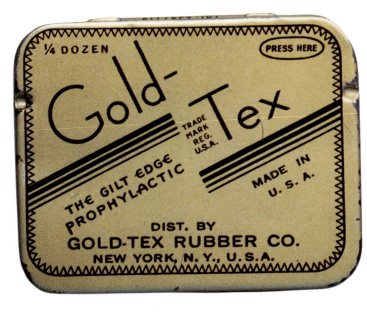

Gold-Tex. Gold-Tex Rubber Company. 2-1/8" x 1-5/8". $350.00.

Hercules (#41). Robert J. Pierce, Inc.
2-1/8" x 1-5/8". $700.00.

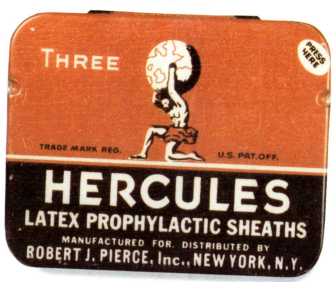

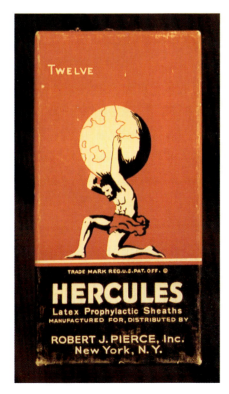

Hercules (cardboard), one dozen. Robert J. Pierce, Inc. 2-3/8" x 5-1/2". $100.00.

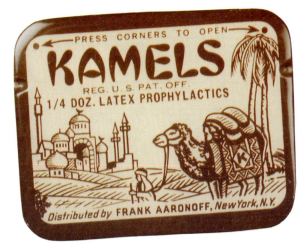

Kamels (# 41), front. Frank Aaronoff. 2-1/8" x 1-5/8". $150.00.

Kamels, back.

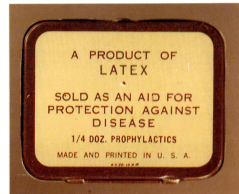

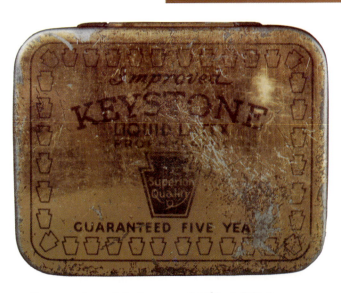

Keystone. Stowall & Company. 2-1/8" x 1-5/8". Rare.

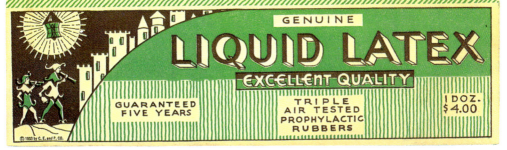

Liquid Latex (paper), Dozen. 9" x 2-1/2".
Manufacturer unknown. $25.00.

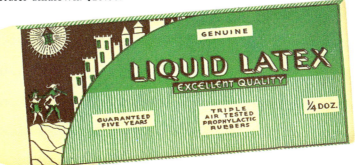

Liquid Latex (paper), 1/4 Dozen. 4-3/4"
x 2". Manufacturer unknown. $20.00.

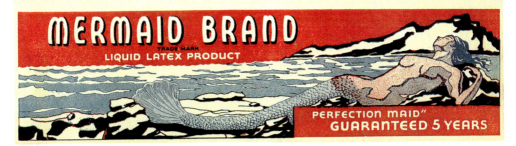

Mermaid (paper) Dozen. 9" x 2-1/2". Manufacturer unknown. $25.00.

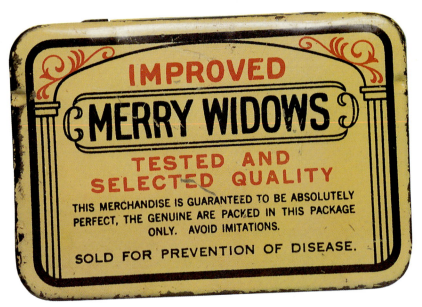

Merry Widows, Improved, front. Manufacturer unknown. 2-5/8" x 1-3/4". Rare.

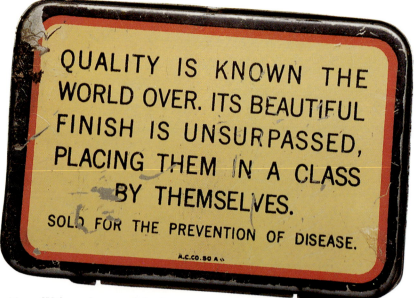

Merry Widows, Improved, back.

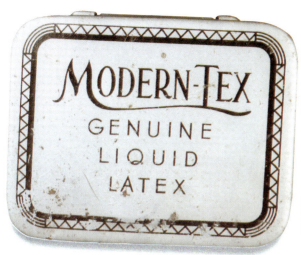

Modern-Tex. Modern
Distributing Company.
2-1/8" x 1-5/8". $100.00.

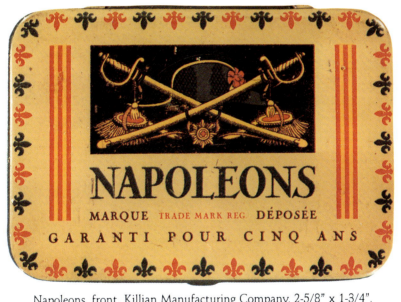

Napoleons, front. Killian Manufacturing Company. 2-5/8" x 1-3/4".
$225.00. They were also made in a World War II version, having a
hinged lid paper packet, with the same front design but in English.

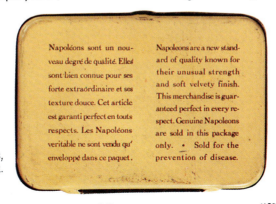

Napoleons,
back.

Napoléons sont un nouveau degré de qualité. Elles sont bien connue pour ses forte extraordinaire et ses texture douce. Cet article est garanti perfect en touts respects. Les Napoléons veritable ne sont vendu qu' enveloppé dans ce paquet.

Napoleons are a new standard of quality known for their unusual strength and soft velvety finish. This merchandise is guaranteed perfect in every respect. Genuine Napoleons are sold in this package only. • Sold for the prevention of disease.

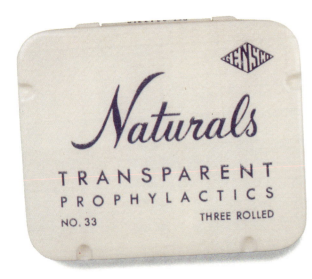

Naturals. Schaeffer
Products Company, Inc.
2-1/4" x 1-3/.4". Rare.
From the same company
that gave us the rare Blue
Goose. So natural it's
flesh colored!

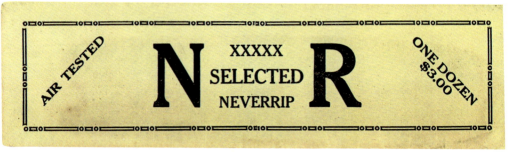

Never Rip (paper), Dozen. 2-1/2" x 8-5/8". Manufacturer unknown. $10.00.

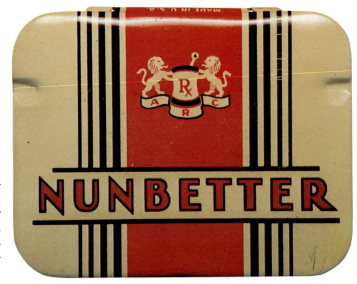

Nunbetter
(# 41), front.
Arrow Rubber
Corporation.
2-1/8" x 1-5/8".
Rare.

¼ DOZEN

NUNBETTER

IS A GENUINE LATEX PRODUCT.
THIN, STRONG AND AIR-TESTED.
FOR YOUR PROTECTION ASK
FOR THEM BY NAME AT YOUR
DRUGGIST.

DISTRIBUTED BY

ARROW RUBBER CORP.
NEW YORK, N. Y.

PRINTED IN U.S.A.

Nunbetter, back.

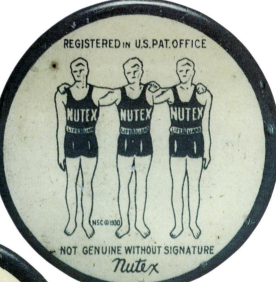

Nutex Lifeguards, front. Nutex Sales Company. 1-1/2" round. Rare. This little gem, dated 1930, is not only a one-of-a-kind, but the only known round rubber tin of its size - 1-1/2" diameter instead of the usual 1-5/8".

REGISTERED IN U.S. PAT. OFFICE

NUTEX NUTEX NUTEX
LIFE GUARD LIFE GUARD LIFE GUARD

NSC©1930

NOT GENUINE WITHOUT SIGNATURE
Nutex

NUTEX
LIFE-GUARDS
ARE DESIGNED

To guard the very life of a nation against the contraction of venereal diseases. The Little Lifeguards here-in contained have been tested in the most exacting way and have been found to be in perfect condition. They are made from the purest latex rubber, air-tested and guaranteed against all imperfections, by the

NUTEX SALES CO.
2003 FAIRMOUNT AVE.
PHILA. PA.

ACME CAN CO

Nutex Lifeguards, back.

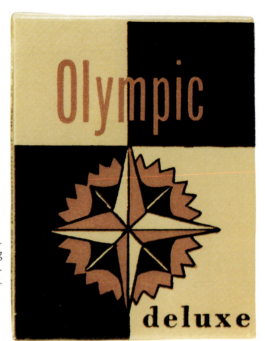

Olympic (paper).
Olympic Vending
Company. 2" x 1-1/2".
$5.00.

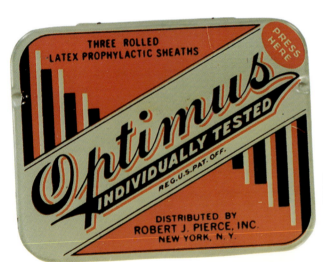

Optimus, front. Robert
J. Pierce, Inc. 2-1/8" x
1-5/8".$125.00

Optimus,
back.

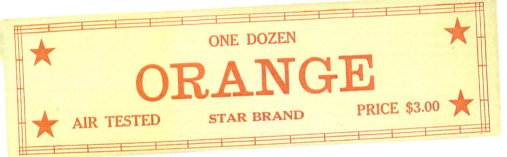

Orange Star Brand (paper), Dozen. 2-1/2" x 9".
Manufacturer unknown. **$10.00.**

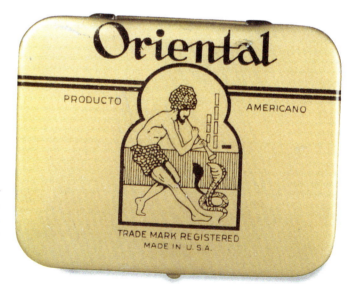

Oriental. Manu-
facturer unknown.
2-1/8" x 1-5/8".
Rare.

47   ORIENTAL

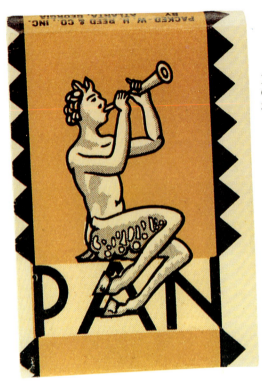

Pan (paper). W.H. Reed &
Company. 1-7/16" x 2-1/8".
$5.00

Pan (paper), one gross.
W.H. Reed & Company.
10" x 4-1/2". $20.00

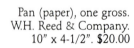

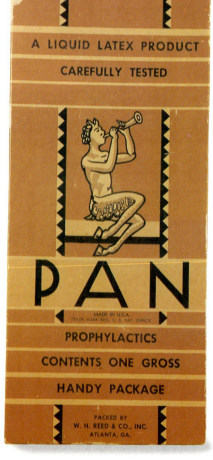

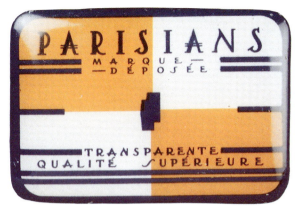

Parisians. Dean Rubber Manufacturing Company. 2-5/8" x 1-3/4". Rare.

PARISIENS—EST FABRIQUÉ DE MATIERES DOUCES ET SURFINES. PAR UN NOVEAU PROCEDE PARISIENS ATTEINT UNE SECURITE ABSOLUE ET NE PEUT ÊTRE SURPASSÉ EN BEAUTE ET QUALITE. LES VRAIS PARISIENS SONT VENDUS EN PAQUET SEULEMENT.

PARISIANS ARE MADE OF THE FINEST QUALITY MATERIAL. BY A NEW PROCESS WHICH GIVES A FINISHED PRODUCT OF UNSURPASSED BEAUTY AND STRENGTH. THIS MERCHANDISE IS GUARANTEED TO BE PERFECT IN EVERY DETAIL. GENUINE PARISIANS ARE SOLD IN THIS CONTAINER ONLY.

SOLD EXCLUSIVELY IN DRUG STORES
DEAN RUBBER MFG. CO.
NORTH KANSAS CITY. MO.

Parisians, back.

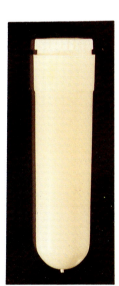

Parisians, (plastic & metal), product. 1-7/8" x 1/2". $25.00.

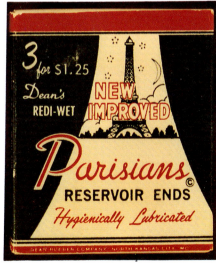

Parisians (paper). Dean Rubber Manufacturing Company. 2-1/8" x 1-7/8". $25.00

49

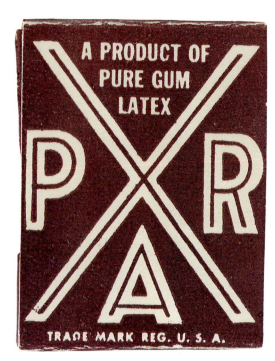

Par-X (paper). Chandler Distributors. 1-7/16" x 2-1/16". $5.00

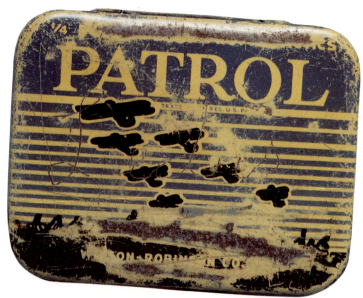

Above & opposite page top:
Patrol. Wilson-Robinson Company, Inc. 2-1/8" x 1-5/8". Rare. These are the only two known examples of the Patrol. It's clear someone who owned the one above deliberately scratched out the words "1/4 dozen prophylactics" and, just to make sure the tin's contents were absolutely untraceable, even rubbed out the company name. A war scene is O.K., but an act of love¿ Heaven forbid! What we have here is a rare, valuable tin destroyed in one fell puritanical swoop! Now that's a sin!

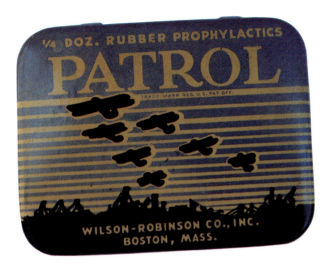

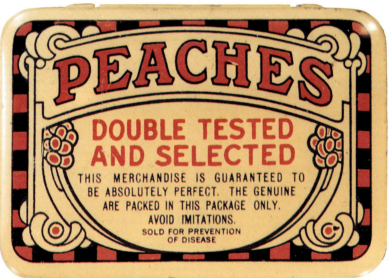

Above:
Peaches, front. Manufacturer unknown. 2-5/8" x 1-3/4". $650.00. There is an "Improved Peaches" of which we could get no photo.

Left:
Peaches, back.

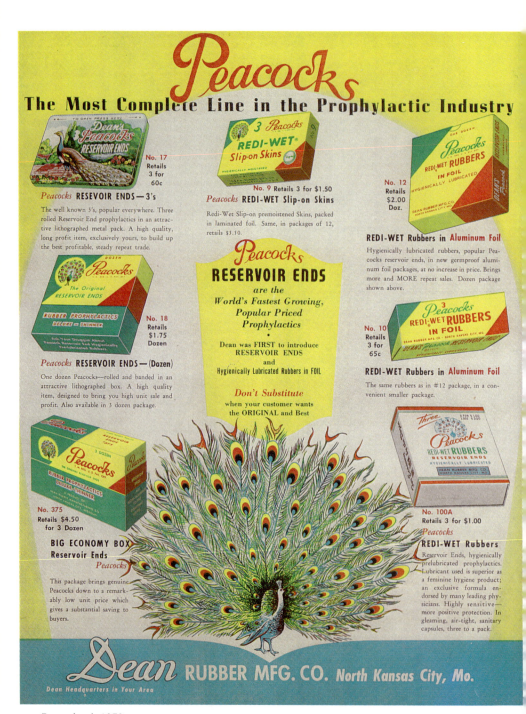

Peacock ad, 1950s.

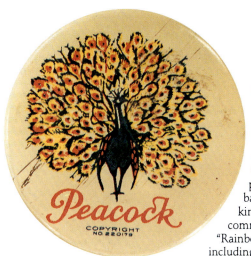

Peacock, copyright 220,179, front. Dean Rubber Manufacturing Company. 1-5/8" round. $150.00. Original U.S. Copyright 220,179 was accepted in 1929 from W.R. Adefsperger. There is another U.S. Copyright 626,562. Dean Rubber Company was the only firm to offer premiums such as bill clips, tape measures, ballpoint pens and mechanical pencils (the kind you put lead in). Dean made the most common "Ultrex Platinum" to the rare "Rainbow" in a huge variety of packaging including tin, paper, foil and plastic.

Peacock, back.

Demand Peacocks. Every one is given a rigid inspection by manufacturer, guaranteed to be perfect. Peacocks are the best quality made by Dean Rubber Co. and are not perfumed to kill kerosene odor as cheaper grades are. Peacocks will not irritate, sold by druggists only.

DEAN RUBBER MFG. CO.
North Kansas City, Mo.
SOLD FOR PREVENTION OF DISEASE ONLY.

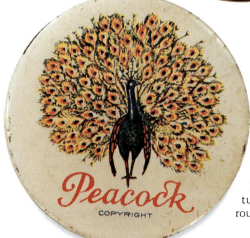

Peacock, copyright (no text on back). Dean Rubber Manufacturing Company. 1-5/8" round. $150.00.

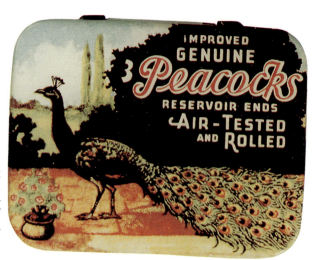

Peacocks, Air-Tested & Rolled, Reservoir Ends. Dean Rubber Manufacturing Company. 2-1/8" x 1-5/8". $100.00.

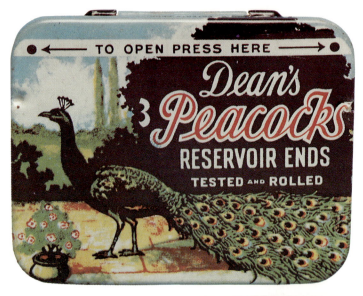

Peacocks, Tested & Rolled, (# 41), Reservoir Ends, front. 2-1/8" x 1-5/8". Dean Rubber Manufacturing Company. $100.00.

Peacocks, Tested & Rolled, (# 41), back.

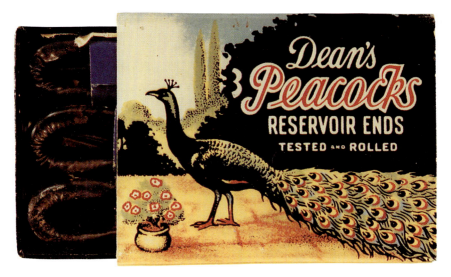

Peacocks, Tested & Rolled (paper shell & slide), World War II era. Dean Rubber Manufacturing Company. 2-1/4" x 1-11/16". $25.00.

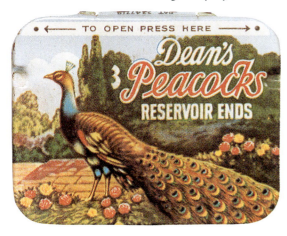

Peacocks, Reservoir Ends, (# 41), number 17, front. Dean Rubber Manufacturing Company. 2-1/8" x 1-5/8". $30.00.

Peacocks, Reservoir Ends, (# 41), number 17, back.

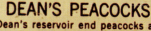

DEAN'S PEACOCKS
Dean's reservoir end peacocks are tested on new, modern equipment for your protection.
Exclusively a drug store item.
An aid in preventing venereal diseases.

THE DEAN RUBBER MFG. COMPANY
NORTH KANSAS CITY, MO.
Registered U. S. Patent No. 220179
Made in U. S. A.

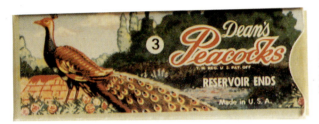

Peacocks (paper), number DF 17. Dean Rubber Manufacturing Company. 2-7/8" x 1". $15.00.

Peacocks, Redi-wet, (paper), number 10. Dean Rubber Manufacturing Company. 2-7/8" x 1". $15.00.

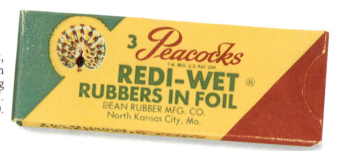

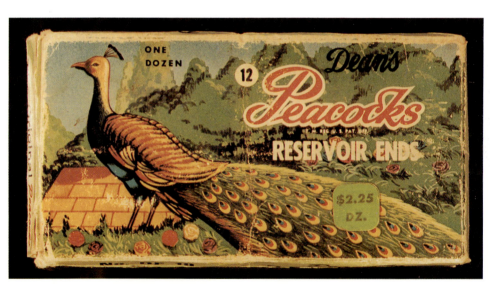

Peacocks (paper), One Dozen, number DF 19. Dean Rubber Manufacturing Company. 4-7/8" x 2-3/8". $25.00.

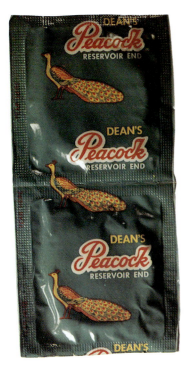

Peacocks (foil),
contents of DF 19.

Peacocks, Redi-wet, (foil),
contents of number 12.

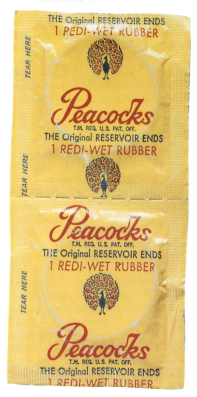

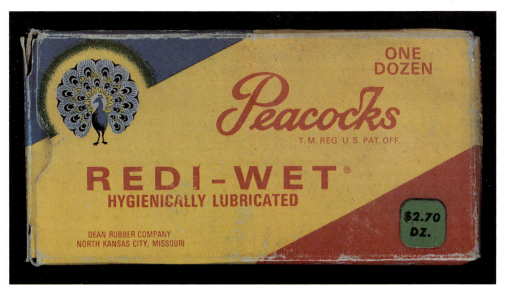

Peacocks, Redi-wet, (paper), One Dozen, No. 12. Copyright 626,563.
Dean Rubber Manufacturing Company. 4-7/8" x 2-3/8". $25.00.

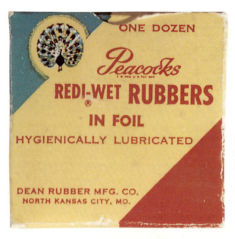

Peacocks, Redi-wet, (paper)
One Dozen, No. 12. Dean
Rubber Manufacturing
Company. 2-3/4" x 2-3/4".
$25.00.

Peacocks (paper),
Dozen, number 18.
Dean Rubber
Manufacturing
Company. 2-5/8" x
1-3/4". $25.00.

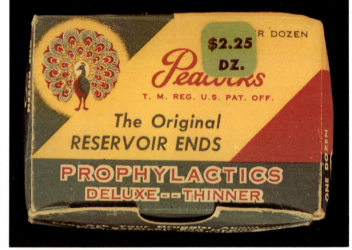

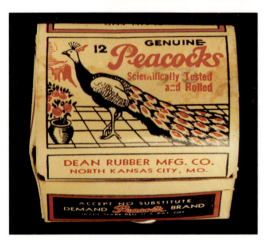

Peacocks (paper) dozen,
trunk, black and white.
Dean Rubber Manufactur-
ing Company. 2" x 1-5/8"
x 1-5/8". $25.00.

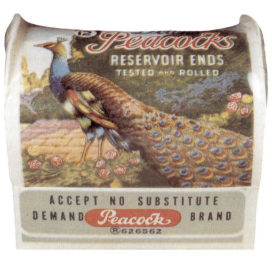

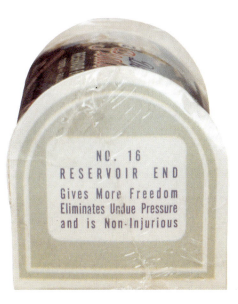

Peacocks (paper) dozen, color trunk.
Dean Rubber Manufacturing Company.
2" x 1-5/8" x 1". $35.00.

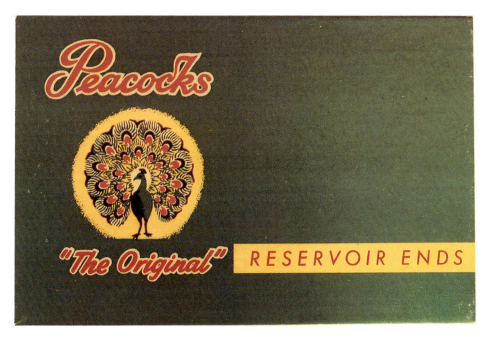

Peacocks (paper), one gross, number 17. Dean Rubber
Manufacturing Company. 6-7/8" x 4-1/2" x 2-1/16". $10.00.

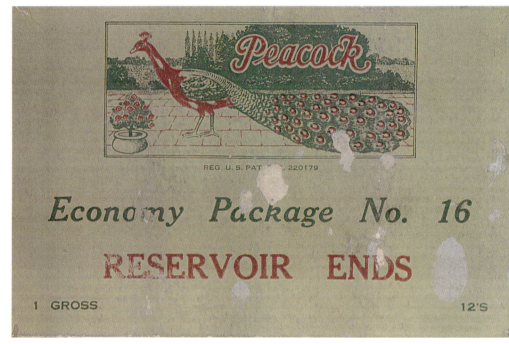

Peacocks (paper), 1 Gross, No. 16. Dean Rubber
Manufacturing Company. 5" x 7-13/16". $10.00.

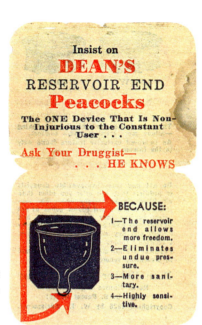

Insist on
DEAN'S
RESERVOIR END
Peacocks

**The ONE Device That Is Non-
Injurious to the Constant
User . . .**

**Ask Your Druggist—
. . . HE KNOWS**

BECAUSE:

1—The reservoir end allows more freedom.

2—Eliminates undue pressure.

3—More sanitary.

4—Highly sensitive.

Peacocks paper insert (front).

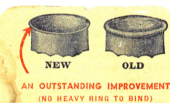

NEW   **OLD**

AN OUTSTANDING IMPROVEMENT
(NO HEAVY RING TO BIND)

This new ring prevents binding or choking
—allows more freedom—more comfort.
An improved exclusive feature found only
in the famous

DEAN PRODUCTS

Do not buy from irresponsible druggists
or peddlers that will offer you other than
air-blown tested merchandise. The majority of peddlers sell rubber goods at cut
prices because they sell throw outs and
seconds. Be certain that the rubber
devices you buy carry the trade-mark of
a reputable rubber goods manufacturer.
Peacocks are all air-blown tested—an aid
in preventing venereal disease.

Dean Rubber Mfg. Company
North Kansas City, Missouri
(Reg. U. S. Patent Office)
Copyrighted 1926 by W. R. Adelsperger.

Peacocks paper insert (back 1).

PROTECT YOUR HEALTH

When a customer purchases a prophylactic, he certainly is buying what
he thinks will give him COMPLETE
protection—and rightly so. It seems
to us the best guide for a customer
to follow to protect his confidence is
to purchase a WELL-KNOWN tried
and proven brand.

PEACOCKS

are manufactured and carefully
tested on the most modern up-to-
date equipment known to the industry—carrying a guarantee backed by
a company who for twenty years has
safeguarded its customers' health
through constant vigilance over its
products—popularizing the RESERVOIR END PEACOCK—a great
HEALTH feature. DEMAND THE
ORIGINAL PEACOCK RESERVOIR END PROPHYLACTIC
FROM YOUR DRUGGIST!

Have you ever tried PEACOCK
REDI-WET SKINS? If you prefer a
natural skin prophylactic—ask your
druggist for DEAN'S PEACOCK
REDI-WET SKINS—pre-moistened
—ready for instant use—no wetting
—no bother—no delay. Another
ORIGINAL improvement by

DEAN RUBBER MFG. COMPANY
North Kansas City, Missouri
Reg. U. S. Patent Office
Copyright 1926 by
W. R. Adelsperger

Peacocks paper insert (back 2).

"IMPORTANT READ"

"LUBRICATION NOT IRRITATION"

"Peacocks" Rediwet Rubbers in foil with the original reservoir end Health feature. Lubricated to perfection with a superior high quality Feminine Hygiene Jelly, suitable to the Rubber. Non-injurious to the most constant user.

- Promotes greater sensitivity
- Reduces friction and strain
- Increases safety, makes prophylactics ready for instant use.
- An aid in the prevention of both venereal disease and trichomonas vaginalis.

Ask for
"Peacocks Rediwet"
The Original in Foil
ACCEPT NO SUBSTITUTE

Sold Exclusively in Drug Stores. "Peacocks" . . . a Brand Name of Distinction.

Peacocks, Redi-wet,
paper insert, yellow.

ALL
rubbers should be
lubricated
DEAN'S PEACOCK REDI-WET RUBBERS
are properly lubricated
Ready for Instant Use
Dean Rubber Manufacturing Co.
North Kansas City, Mo.

Peacocks, Redi-wet,
paper insert, red (front).

LUBRICATION
not
IRRITATION
ask for
DEAN'S PEACOCK REDI-WET RUBBERS
scientifically lubricated
ASK YOUR DRUGGIST

Peacocks, Redi-wet,
paper insert, red, (back).

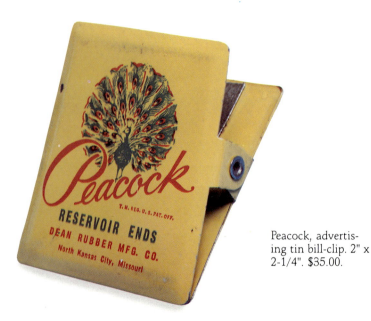

Peacock, advertising tin bill-clip. 2" x 2-1/4". $35.00.

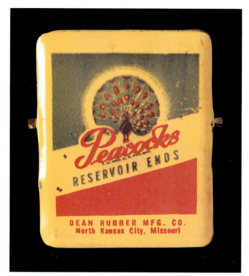

Peacocks, advertising tin bill-clip. 2" x 2-1/4". $35.00.

Peacocks keychain (metal), front. 1-5/8" x 3/4". Rare.

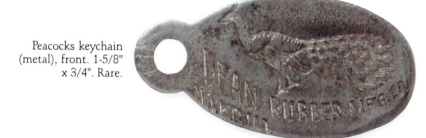

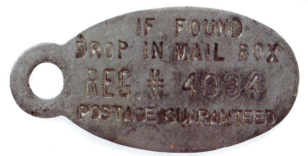

Peacocks keychain, back. If you dropped it in the mailbox, where would it go? and what would they send?

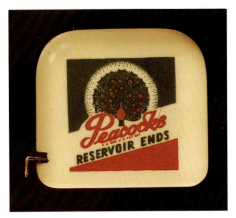

Peacocks plastic & metal tape measure, front. $35.00.

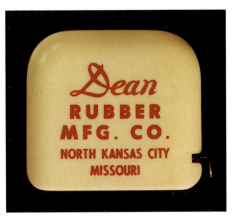

Peacocks tape measure, back.

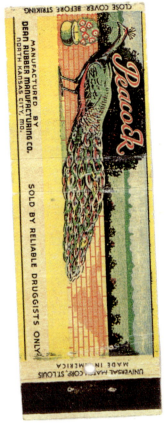

Peacock (paper) matchbook (front). $20.00.

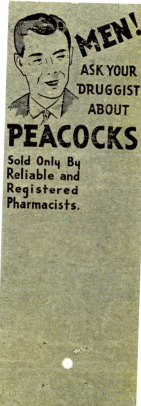

Peacock (paper) matchbook (back).

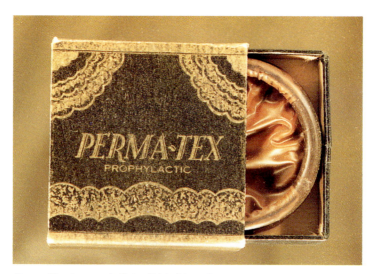

Perma-Tex (paper shell & slide). Manufacturer
unknown. 1-11/16" x 1-11/16".

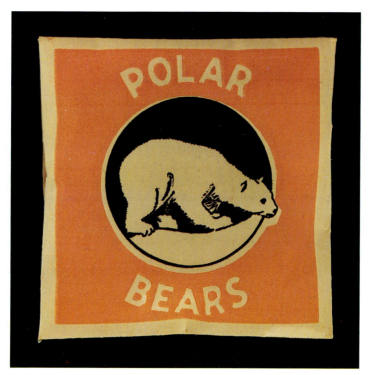

Polar Bears, (paper). Sterling Rubber
Company. 2-1/4" x 2-1/4". $15.00.

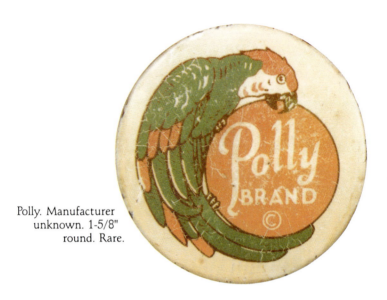

Polly. Manufacturer unknown. 1-5/8" round. Rare.

FOR YOUR PROTECTION— DEMAND POLLY BRAND

POLLY BRAND is double air tested, assuring you no holes and a 100% perfect piece of goods.

POLLY BRAND is made of the pure milk from the rubber tree, and is free from any chemical compounds, gasoline or naphthas.

POLLY BRAND is cured in boiling water; therefore, free from odors, and most sanitary.

POLLY BRAND is less than half in weight of gasoline made goods, yet they are more than 100% stronger in tensile strength.

POLLY BRAND goods are guaranteed against deterioration for 5 years.

POLLY BRAND

Polly, (paper) ad insert and warning insert.

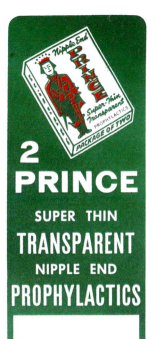

Prince, decal for machine. 17" x 3".

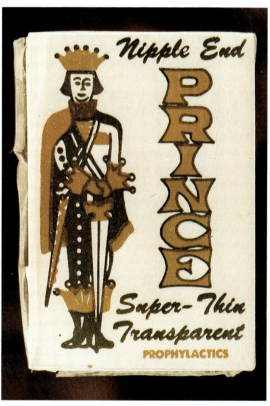

Prince, (paper). Circle Rubber Corporation. 2-1/4" x 1-1/2". $5.00.

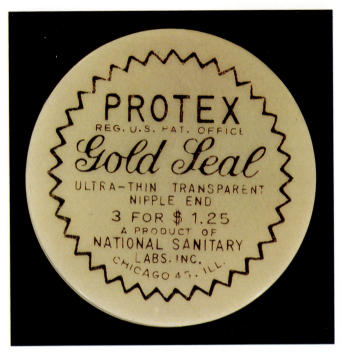

Protex Gold Seal. National Sanitary
Labs, Inc.. 1-3/4" round. $15.00.

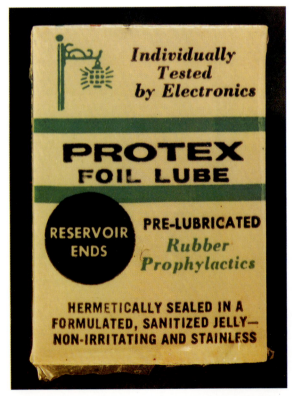

Protex Foil Lube,
(paper), number
125. National
Sanitary Sales, Inc.
2-1/16" x 1-1/2".

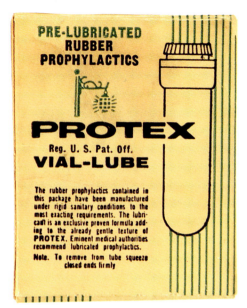

Protex Vial-Lube,
number 100.
National Sanitary
Sales, Inc. 2-1/4"
x 1-3/4". $15.00.

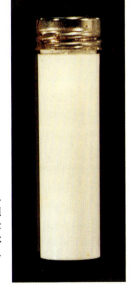

Protex Vial-
Lube, (metal
cap, plastic
tube). 2-1/4" x
5/8".

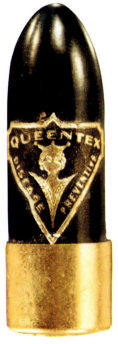

Queen-tex (metal cap,
plastic body) lipstick
shape. Manufacturer
unknown. 2" x 5/8".
$10.00. Meant to look
like a lipstick tube for
milady's purse.

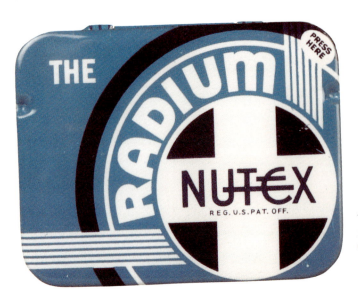

The Radium Nutex,
front. Nutex Sales
Company. 2-1/8" x
1-5/8". $200.00.

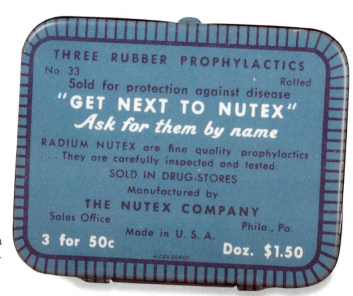

The Radium
Nutex, back.

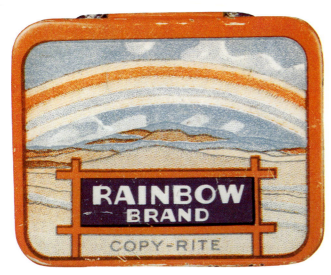

Rainbow. Dean Rubber Manufacturing Company. 2-1/8" x 1-5/8". Rare.

Rainbow, back.

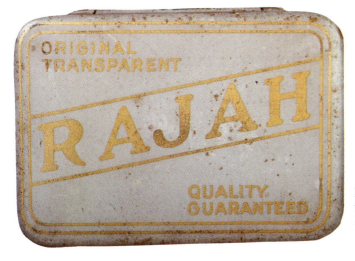

Rajah. Manufacturer unknown. 2-5/8" x 1-3/4". Rare.

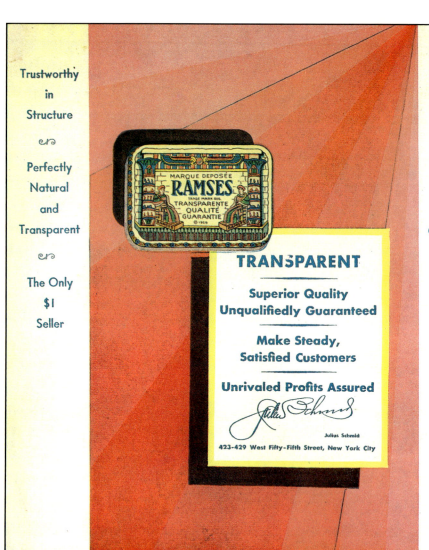

Ramses ad, 1930.

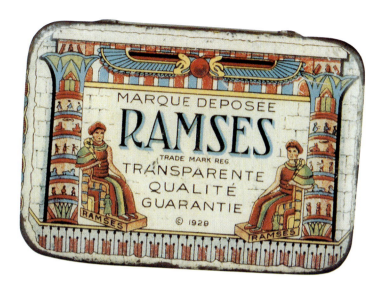

Ramses, copyright 1929 (# 41), front. Julius Schmid, Inc. 2-5/8" x 1-3/4". $225.00. The flagship of the Schmid Company. Just about everything they made had a leaflet telling you why you want to buy "Ramses," though why anyone would name a rubber after a guy who fathered more than two hundred children is a puzzle. In the 19th century Julius Schmid's original business was sausage skin and membrane bottle seal maker. His first factory was on Long Island in 1882. In 1888 he started processing lamb cecum into condoms. According to the U.S. Copyright office, the first use of "Ramses" as a brand name was March 19, 1926. The Copyright 247,841 was granted on October 29, 1928. Julius Schmid also registered "Ramses" as a brand name for vaginal diaphragms and vaginal jelly. There are "Ramses Diaphragms" in tin, which are very hard to find without rust. Ramses is also a cigarette brand, starting around World War I and still sold today.

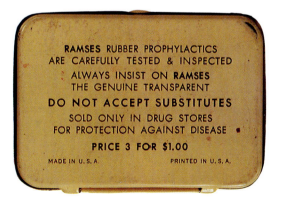

Ramses, copyright 1929, back.

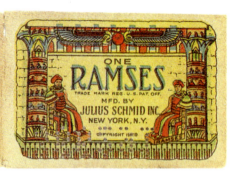

Ramses, copyright
1929 (paper),
envelope.

Ramses copyright 1929
(paper), insert ad.

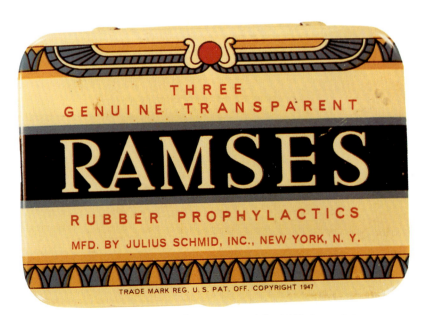

Ramses, copyright 1947, front. Julius
Schmid, Inc.. 2-5/8" x 1-3/4". $200.00.

RAMSES RUBBER PROPHYLACTICS
ARE CAREFULLY TESTED & INSPECTED

ALWAYS INSIST ON **RAMSES**
THE GENUINE TRANSPARENT

DO NOT ACCEPT SUBSTITUTES

SOLD ONLY IN DRUG STORES
FOR PROTECTION AGAINST DISEASE

PRICE 3 FOR $1.00

MADE IN U.S.A.   PRINTED IN U.S.A.

Ramses, copyright 1947, back.

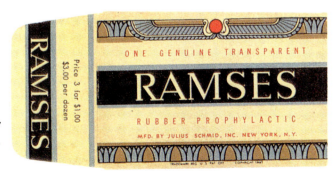

TO BETTER preserve their unique qualities of transparency and glossy finish, RAMSES are packed in unrolled form. By the simple process of placing the rubber on two fingers, spread to create tension, it may be rolled with ease for convenient use. See illustrations to the right.

Ask for RAMSES by name.
Accept no substitute.

Manufactured by
JULIUS SCHMID, INC.
NEW YORK 19, N. Y.

Sold in Drug Stores Only —
For Protection against Disease.

PLACE THE RUBBER ON
TWO FINGERS. SPREAD
TO CREATE TENSION.

ROLL UPWARD WITH
OTHER HAND. (AS
SHOWN ABOVE).

Ramses copyright 1947
(paper), insert ad.

Ramses copyright 1947
(paper), envelope.

ONE GENUINE TRANSPARENT

RAMSES

RUBBER PROPHYLACTIC

MFD. BY JULIUS SCHMID, INC. NEW YORK, N.Y.

RAMSES

Price 3 for $1.00
$3.00 per dozen

RAMSES

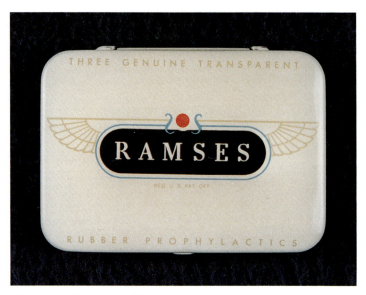

Ramses (white). Julius Schmid, Inc.
2-5/8" x 1-3/4". $200.00.

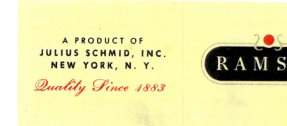

A PRODUCT OF
JULIUS SCHMID, INC.
NEW YORK, N. Y.
Quality Since 1883

RAMSES

Ramses (paper)
insert ad, front.
Found in "Sheik"
tins .

Ramses
(paper) insert
ad, back.

Attention!

Have you ever tried Ramses? There are several types and finishes of rubber prophylactics from which you can choose, but only one Ramses —the thin, strong, durable and exclusively transparent product with such a glossy, soft surface smoothness that distinguishes it as being the really 'different' prophylactic. If you want the ultimate in a satisfactory product, ask your druggist for Ramses the next time you buy. They are available in handy tins of 3—or in the economy package of 12.

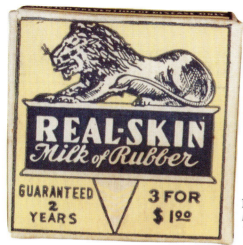

Real Skin (paper).
Manufacturer unknown.
1-3/4" x 1-5/8". $20.00.

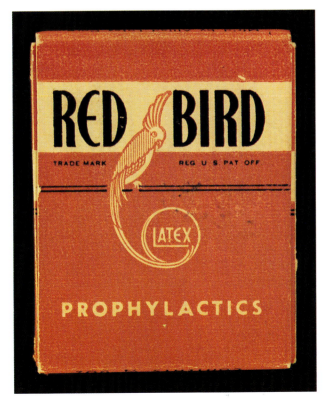

Red Bird (paper). Allied Latex Sales Division. 2-1/16" x
1-5/8". $20.00. This paper box of one dozen was a gift
from a friend. He was cleaning his basement and noticed
a loose brick in the furnace stack. When he removed the
brick, behind it were two boxes of one dozen.

RED BIRD

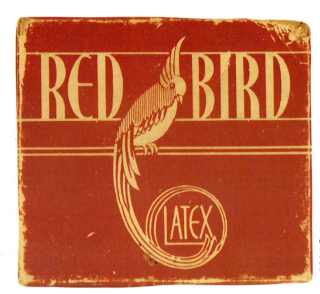

Red Bird (paper), one dozen, outside. Allied Latex Sales Division. 2-3/4" x 2-7/16".

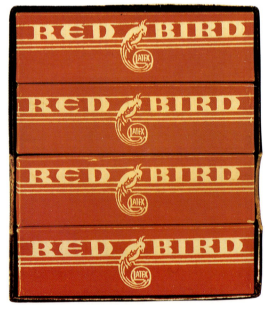

Red Bird (paper), one dozen, inside.

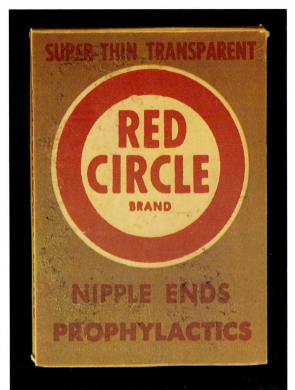

Red Circle (paper). Manufacturer unknown. 2-3/4" x 2-7/16". $10.00.

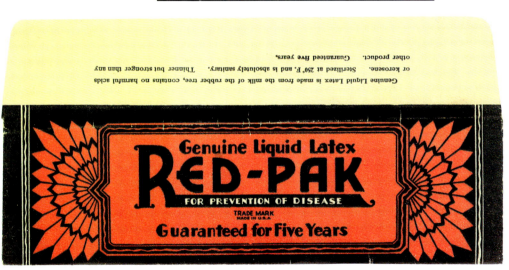

Red-Pak (paper), dozen. Manufacturer unknown. 9" x 2-1/2". $10.00.

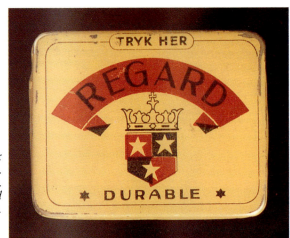

Regard. Manufacturer and country unknown. 2-1/8" x 1-5/8". Rare. *Courtesy of Richard Oatley.*

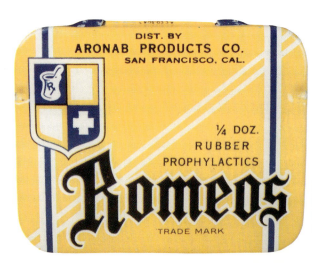

Romeos, (# 41), yellow, front. Killian Manufacturing Company. 2-1/8" x 1-5/8". $150.00.

Romeos, yellow, back.

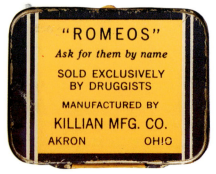

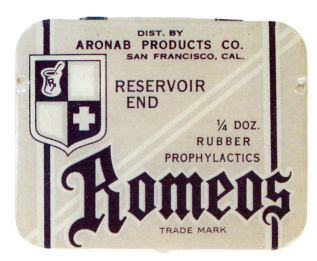

Romeos, (# 41), violet, front. Killian Manufacturing Company. 2-1/8" x 1-5/8". Rare.

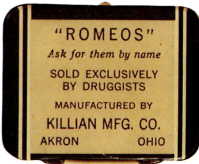

Romeos, violet, back.

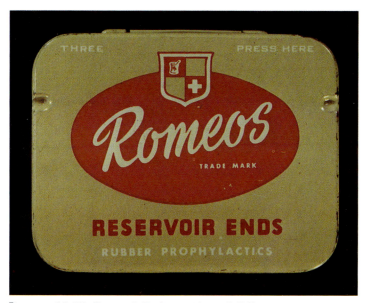

Romeos, (# 41), Reservoir Ends outside oval. Killian Manufacturing Company. 2-1/8" x 1-5/8". $125.00.

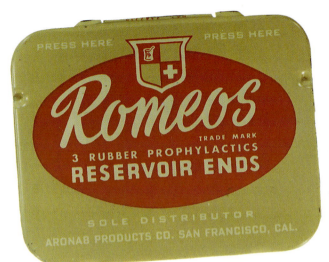

Romeos,(# 41), Reservoir
Ends inside oval, front.
Killian Manufacturing
Company, distributed by
Aronab Products Company.
2-1/8" x 1-5/8". $125.00.

Romeos, Reservoir
Ends-inside oval,
back.

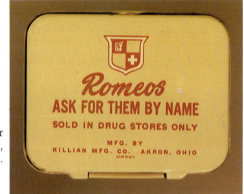

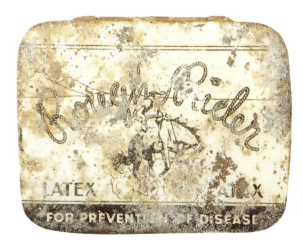

Rough Rider.
International
Distributors. 2-1/8"
x 1-5/8". Rare.

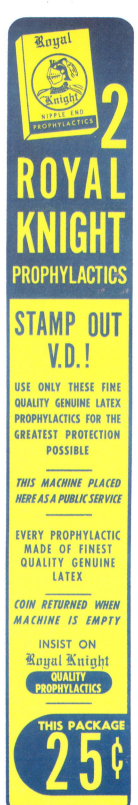

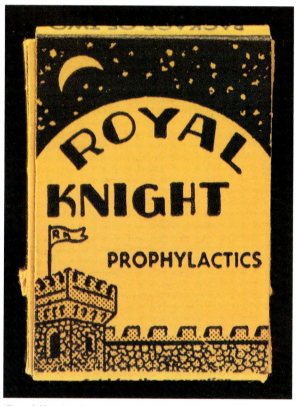

Royal Knight, (paper), castle. Central Sundries, Inc. 2-1/8" x 1-1/2". $45.00.

Royal Knight, decal for machine. Allied Latex Sales Company. 17" x 3-1/4".

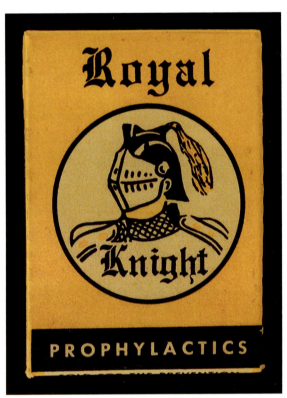

Royal Knight, (paper), knight. Allied Latex
Sales Company. 2-1/4" x 1-1/2". $30.00.

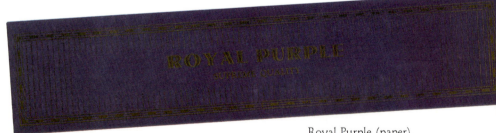

Royal Purple (paper),
dozen. Manufacturer
unknown. 10-1/4" x 2-1/4".
$8.00.

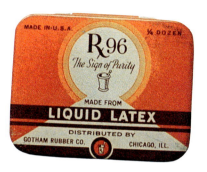

RX 96. Gotham
Rubber Company.
2-1/8" x 1-5/8".
*Courtesy of Michael
Kain. Rare.*

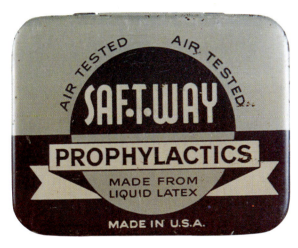

Saf-T-Way, front.
Gotham Rubber
Company. 2-1/8" x
1-5/8". $125.00.

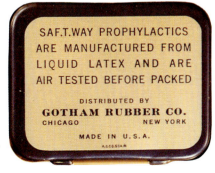

Saf-T-Way, back.

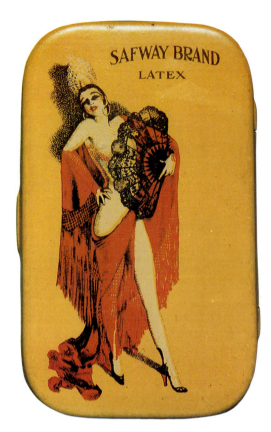

Safway Brand. Manufacturer unknown. 1-5/8" x 2-5/8". Rare. Here's a "variation on Carmen!" Same girl, different brand. We've all seen tins with "go-with" variations of size, design, or color, but a name change is most unusual! This is also the only known rubber tin of its size and with hinges on the left.

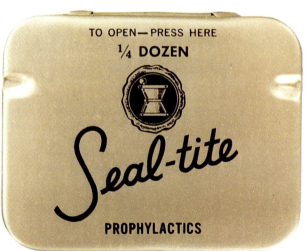

Seal-tite, front. Allied Latex Sales Division. 2-1/8" x 1-5/8". $75.00. There is also a "Seal-Test" rubber tin. Same design, same company. Rare.

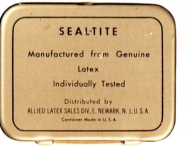

Seal-tite, back.

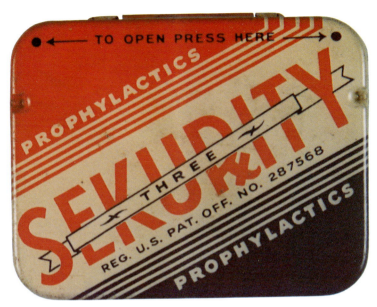

Sekurity, front. Dean Rubber Manufacturing Company. 2-1/8" x 1-5/8". $150.00.

Sekurity, back.

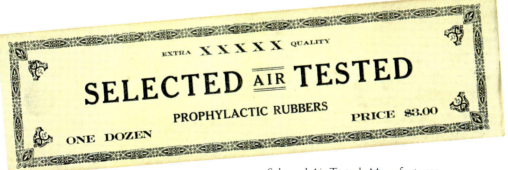

Selected-Air-Tested. Manufacturer unknown. 9" x 2-1/2". $8.00.

SELECTED

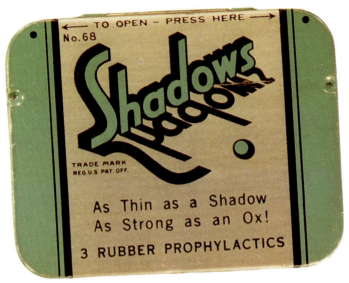

Shadows (# 41), No. 68, front.
Youngs Rubber Corporation.
2-1/8" x 1-5/8". $125.00.

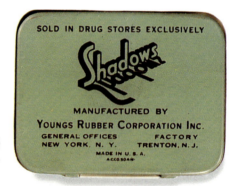

Shadows (# 41)
No. 68, back.

Shadows, (paper) No. 65.
Youngs Rubber Corporation,
Inc. 2-1/8" x 1-5/8". $10.00.

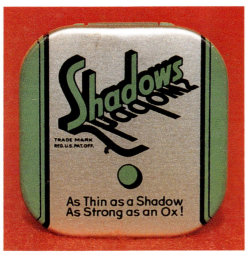

Shadows, square, front. Youngs Rubber
Corporation. 1-5/8" x 1-5/8". $100.00.

Shadows,
square, back.

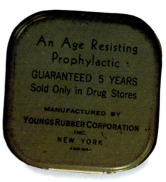

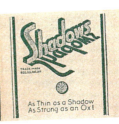

Shadows (paper) insert ad, front.

Shadows insert ad, back.

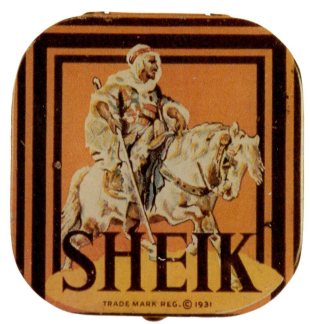

Sheik, square, front.
Julius Schmid, Inc.
1-5/8" x 1-5/8".
$150.00.

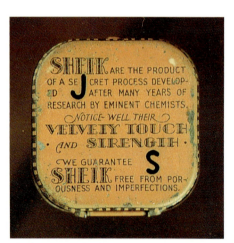

SHEIK ARE THE PRODUCT
OF A SECRET PROCESS DEVELOP-
ED AFTER MANY YEARS OF
RESEARCH BY EMINENT CHEMISTS.
NOTICE WELL THEIR
VELVETY TOUCH
AND STRENGTH
WE GUARANTEE
SHEIK FREE FROM POR-
OUSNESS AND IMPERFECTIONS.

Sheik, square, back.

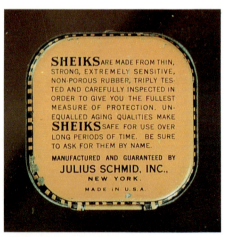

SHEIKS ARE MADE FROM THIN,
STRONG, EXTREMELY SENSITIVE,
NON-POROUS RUBBER, TRIPLY TES-
TED AND CAREFULLY INSPECTED IN
ORDER TO GIVE YOU THE FULLEST
MEASURE OF PROTECTION. UN-
EQUALLED AGING QUALITIES MAKE
SHEIKS SAFE FOR USE OVER
LONG PERIODS OF TIME. BE SURE
TO ASK FOR THEM BY NAME.
MANUFACTURED AND GUARANTEED BY
JULIUS SCHMID, INC.,
NEW YORK.
MADE IN U.S.A.

Sheik, square, back.

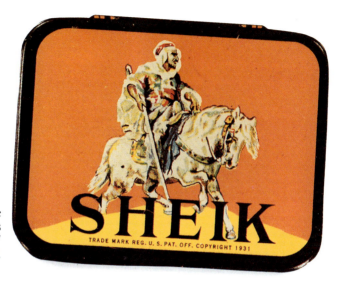

Sheik, with name at bottom. Julius Schmid, Inc. 2-1/8" x 1-5/8". $75.00.

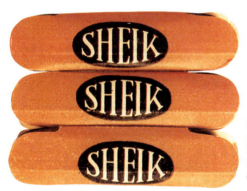

Sheik, (rubber & paper) product, front. U.S. Patent 2,231,254. Only found in Sheik, name on bottom of tin.

Sheik, (rubber & paper) product, back.

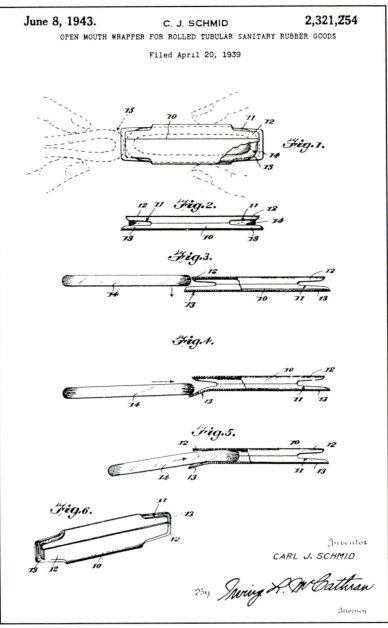

June 8, 1943.   C. J. SCHMID   2,321,254
OPEN MOUTH WRAPPER FOR ROLLED TUBULAR SANITARY RUBBER GOODS

Filed April 20, 1939

Fig.1.

Fig.2.

Fig.3.

Fig.4.

Fig.5.

Fig.6.

Inventor
CARL J. SCHMID

By Irving L. McCathran
Attorney

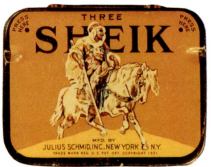

Above:
Illustration from U.S.
Patent 2,321,245.

Left:
Sheik, name at top (# 41).
Julius Schmid, Inc. 2-1/8" x
1-5/8". $60.00.

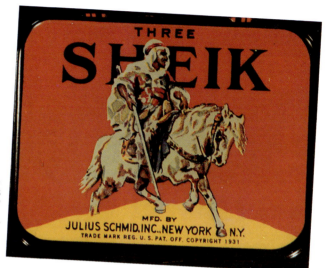

Sheik, name at top, front. Julius Schmid, Inc.. 2-1/8" x 1-5/8". $60.00.

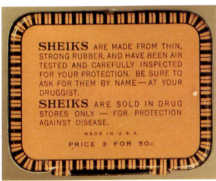

Sheik, name at top, back.

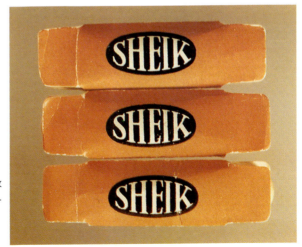

Sheik, (paper & rubber) product.

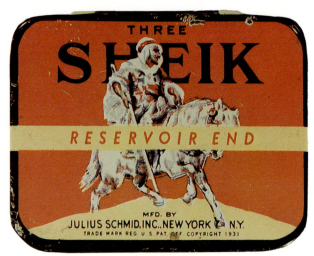

Sheik, Reservoir End, No. 28. Julius Schmid, Inc. 2-1/8" x 1-5/8". $50.00.

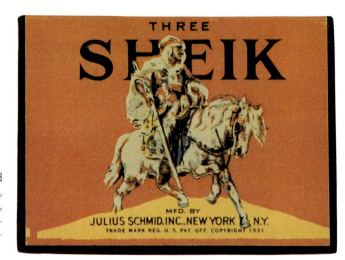

Sheik,(paper, hinged lid) World War II era, front. Julius Schmid, Inc. 2-1/2" x 1-5/8". $25.00.

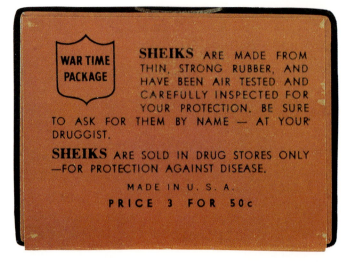

Sheik,(paper, hinged lid), back, marked "War Time Package.".

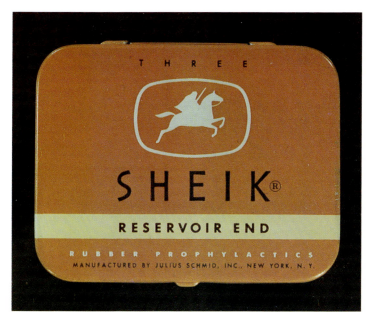

Above:
Sheik, brown, No. 28, front.
Julius Schmid, Inc. 2-1/8" x
1-5/8". $35.00.

Right:
Sheik, brown, No. 28, back.

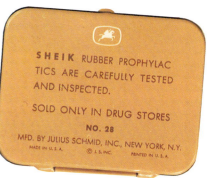

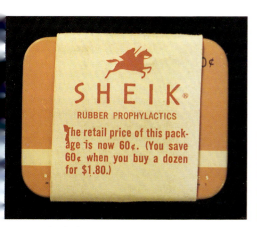

Sheik, brown (with paper wrapper),
No. 28, front. Julius Schmid, Inc. 2-1/8"
x 1-5/8". $50.00.

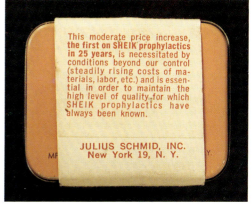

Sheik, brown (with paper
wrapper), No. 28, back.

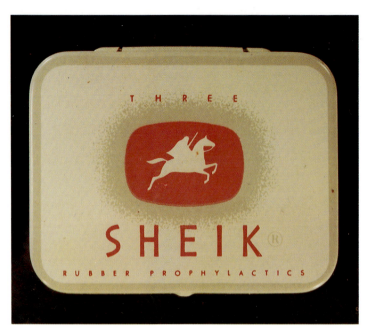

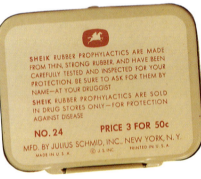

Above:
Sheik, white, No. 24, front.
Julius Schmid, Inc. 2-1/8"
x 1-5/8". $30.00.

Left:
Sheik, white, No. 24, back.

Sheik, (paper & rubber)
product, found in
white tin. U.S. Patent
2,390,900.

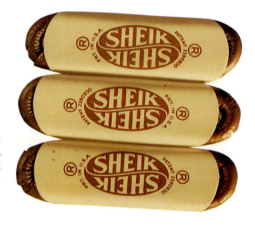

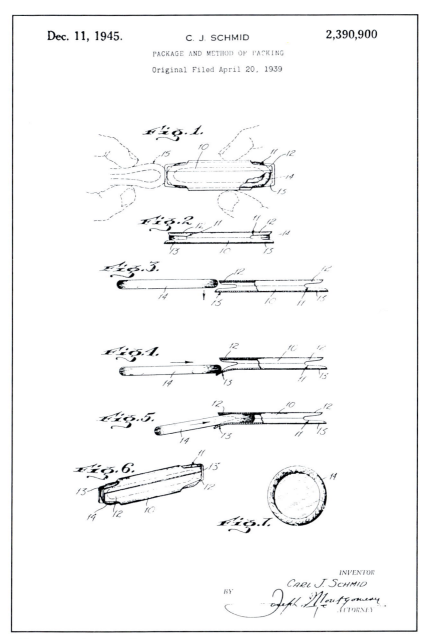

Dec. 11, 1945. C. J. SCHMID 2,390,900

PACKAGE AND METHOD OF PACKING

Original Filed April 20, 1939

INVENTOR

Carl J. Schmid

BY

ATTORNEY

U.S. Patent 2,390,900, illustration.

Insert found in
Sheik tin.

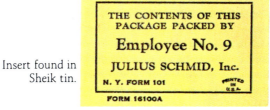

THE CONTENTS OF THIS
PACKAGE PACKED BY

Employee No. 9

JULIUS SCHMID, Inc.

N. Y. FORM 101   PRINTED IN U.S.A.

FORM 16100A

97   SHEIK

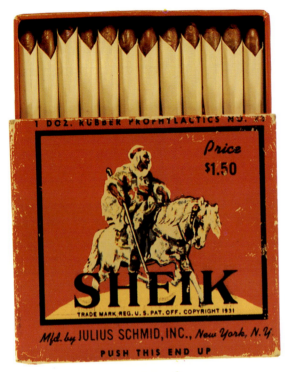

Sheik (paper), One Dozen, No. 23. Julius Schmid, Inc. 2-3/8" x 2-3/16". $25.00.

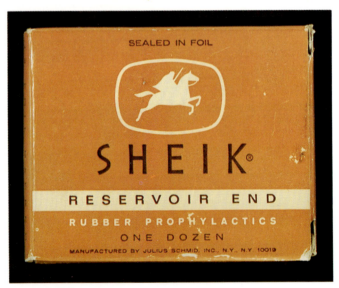

Sheik (paper), One Dozen, No. 29. Julius Schmid, Inc. 2-3/4" x 2-1/4". $20.00.

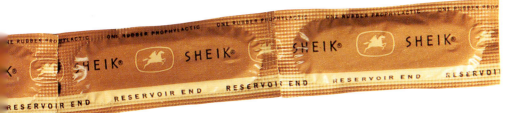

Sheik (foil), product from No. 29.

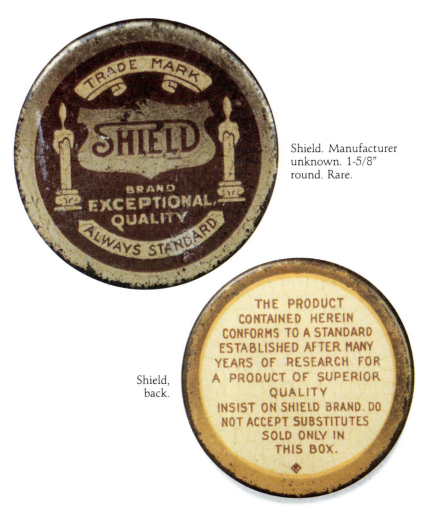

Shield. Manufacturer unknown. 1-5/8" round. Rare.

Shield, back.

SHEILD

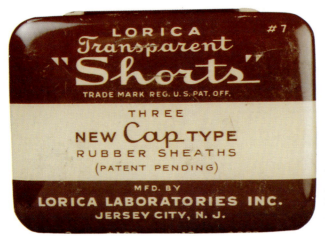

"Shorts." Lorica Laboratories Inc. 2-5/8" x 1-3/4". Rare

"Shorts" (paper), instructions insert.

2

Lubricate outside only with some vegetable lubricant—not Vaseline.

CAUTION

Do not place band as far back as it will go because then there will be nothing to hold it in place and there will be no reservoir left in bag.

1

Nature has provided a GROOVE into which the BAND of the "SHORTS" is designed and intended to fit snugly. Do not place the BAND at any other position than snugly and flatly in the bottom of this GROOVE.

Eliminate trapped air by lifting band slightly and twisting bag.

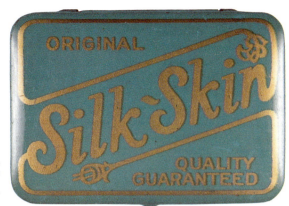

Silk-Skin. Manufacturer unknown. 2-5/8" x 1-3/4". Rare.

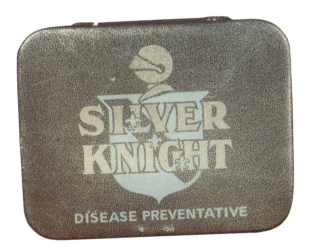

Silver Knight. L.J. McFadden Company. 2-1/8" x 1-5/8". Rare.

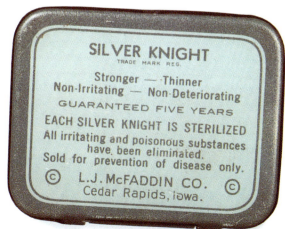

Silver Knight, back.

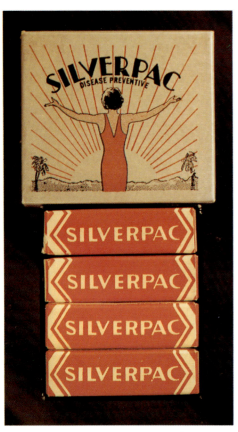

Silverpac (paper) one dozen. Manufacturer
unknown. 2-13/16" x 2-7/16". Rare.
Courtesy of Richard Oatley.

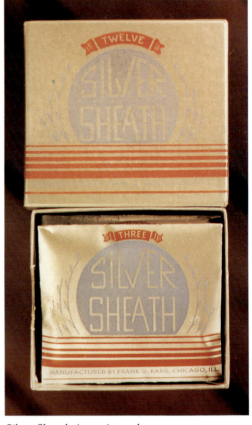

Silver Sheath (paper), twelve .
Frank G. Karg. 2-13/16" x 2-7/16".
Rare. *Courtesy of Richard Oatley.*

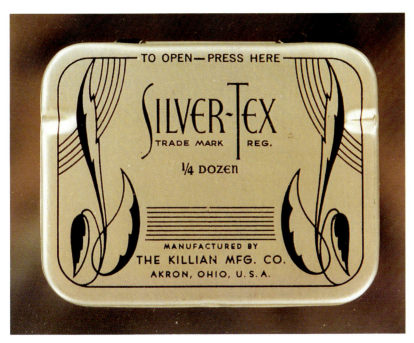

Silver-Tex, (# 41), front. Killian Manufacturing Company. 2-1/8" x 1-5/8". $75.00.

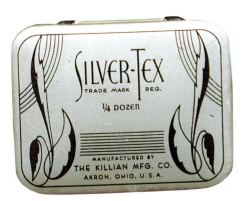

Silver-Tex, front. Killian Manufacturing Company. 2-1/8" x 1-5/8". $75.00.

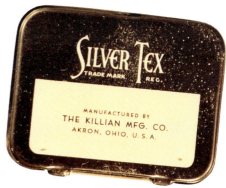

Silver-Tex, back.

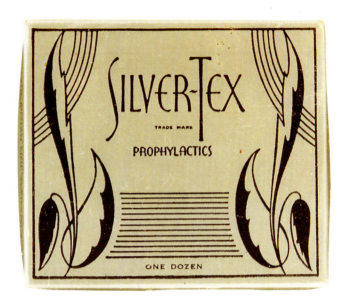

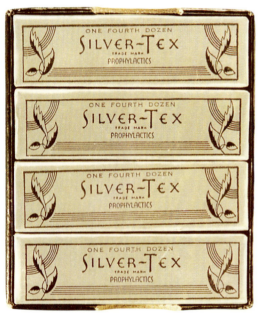

Above:
Silver-Tex, (paper) One Dozen, outside. Killian Manufacturing Company. 2-13/16" x 2-7/16". $15.00.

Left:
Silver-Tex, (paper), one dozen, inside.

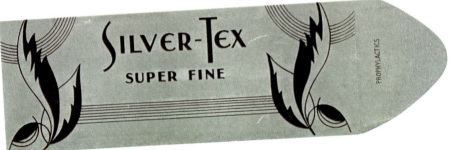

Silver-Tex, 1/4 Dozen, paper envelope. Killian Manufacturing Company. 4-3/4" x 1-3/4". $15.00

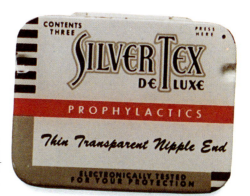

Silver-Tex De-Luxe. Killian
Manufacturing Company.
2-1/8" x 1-5/8". *Courtesy of
Michael Kain. Rare.*

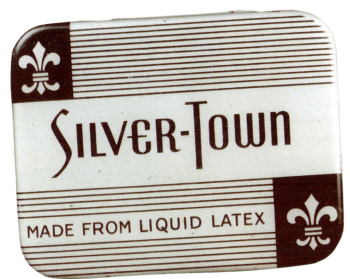

Silver Town, front.
Mayfair Chemical
Corporation. 2-1/8"
x 1-5/8". $125.00.

Silver Town, back.

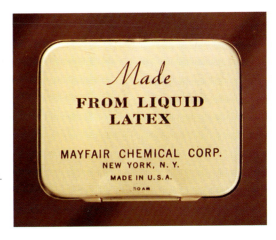

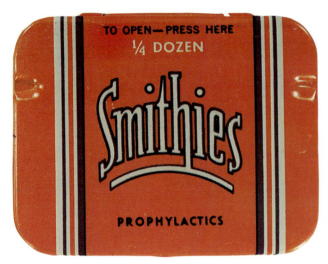

Smithies (# 41),
front. Allen Latex
Sales Division.
2-1/8" x 1-5/8".
Rare.

Smithies,
back.

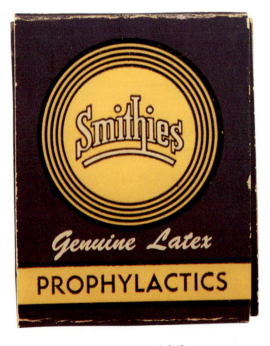

Smithies (paper), blue.
Allied Latex Sales
Division. 2-1/8" x 1-5/8".
$15.00.

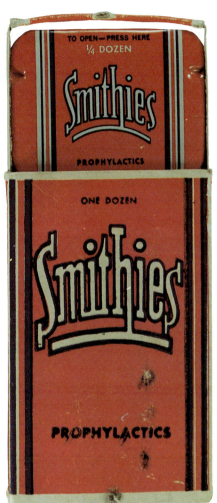

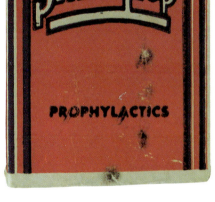

Smithies (paper), One Dozen. Allied Latex Sales Division. Held four tins. 3-9/16" x 2-1/4". $15.00.

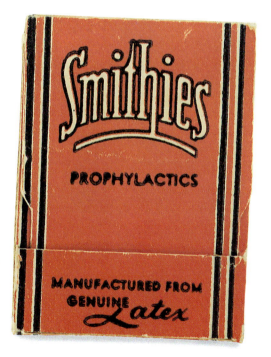

Smithies (paper), orange. Allied Latex Sales Division. 2-1/8" x 1-5/8". $15.00.

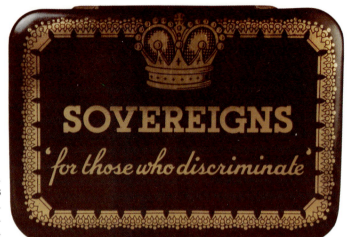

Sovereigns.
Excello Hygienics
Products Corp.
2-5/8" x 1-3/4".
$500.00.

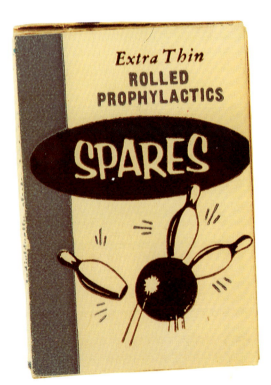

Spares, (paper). National Sanitary
Sales, Inc. 2-1/8" x 1-1/2". $15.00.

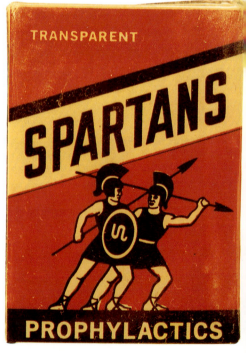

Spartans, (paper). M & M Rubber
Company. 2-1/8" x 1-1/2". $10.00.

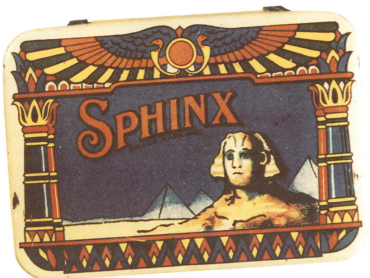

Sphinx, front. Julius Schmid,
Inc. 2-5/8" x 1-3/4". Rare.

Sphinx, back.

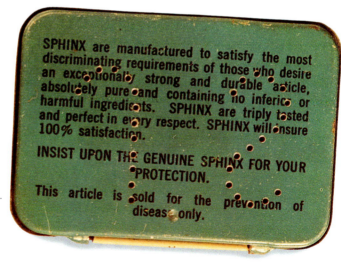

SPHINX are manufactured to satisfy the most discriminating requirements of those who desire an exceptionally strong and durable article, absolutely pure and containing no inferior or harmful ingredients. SPHINX are triply tested and perfect in every respect. SPHINX will ensure 100% satisfaction.

INSIST UPON THE GENUINE SPHINX FOR YOUR PROTECTION.

This article is sold for the prevention of disease only.

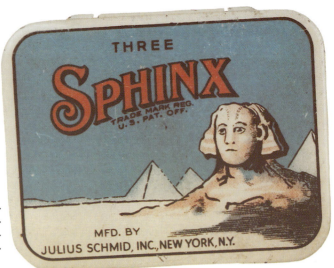

Sphinx, Three, front.
Julius Schmid, Inc.
2-1/8" x 1-5/8".
Rare.

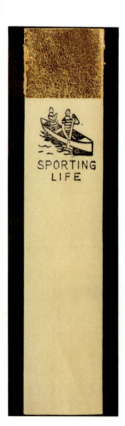

Sphinx, Three, back.

Sporting Life, (paper & foil)
cigarette wrapper, front.
Manufacturer unknown.
$5.00. No one has found one of
these with the product intact.
It is believed that you slipped
it into your cigarette pack.

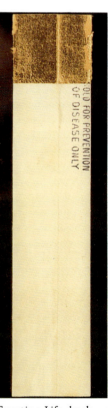

Sporting Life, back.

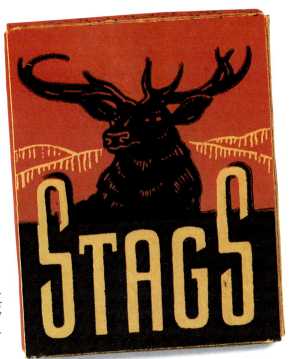

Stags, (paper).
Goodwear Rubber
Company, Inc.. 2-1/8"
x 1-5/8". $25.00.

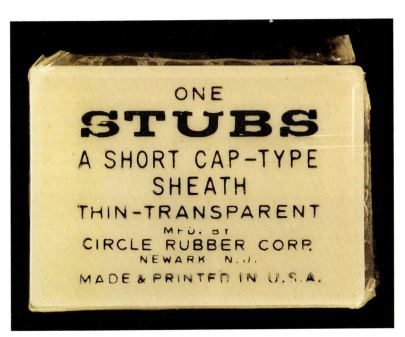

Stubs, (plastic). Circle Rubber
Corporation. 2-1/8" x 1-1/2". $20.00.

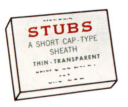

STUBS
A SHORT CAP-TYPE
SHEATH
THIN-TRANSPARENT

GENUINE LATEX
STUBS

A SHORT
CAP TYPE
SHEATH

THIN
TRANSPARENT

MADE IN THE
U.S.A.

COIN RETURNED
WHEN
MACHINE IS
EMPTY

Stubs, decal
for machine.
Circle Rubber
Corporation.
17" x 3-3/4".

THIS PACKAGE
25¢

USE QUARTERS
ONLY

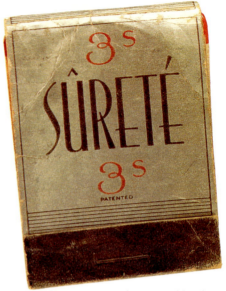

Surete, (paper) faux matchbook,
outside. W.H. Reed $ Company,
Inc. 2-3/8" x 1-13/16". $40.00.

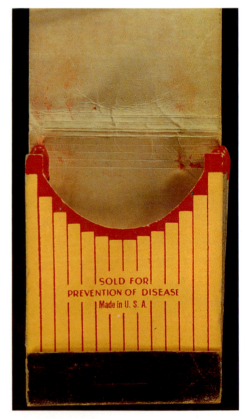

SOLD FOR
PREVENTION OF DISEASE
Made in U. S. A.

Surete, (paper) faux
match book, inside.

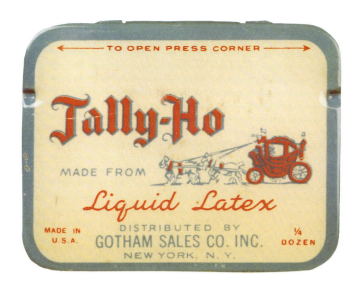

Above:
Tally-Ho, front. Gotham Sales Company, Inc. 2-5/8" x 1-5/8". Rare.

Left:
Tally-Ho, back.

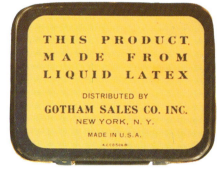

Tetratex, (paper). L.E. Shunk Latex Products, Inc. 2" x 1-5/8". $5.00.

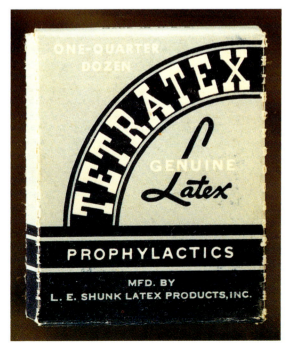

TETRATEX

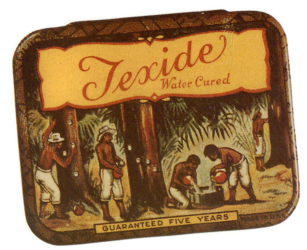

Texide, Guaranteed
Five Years, front.
L.E. Shunk Latex
Products, Inc. 2-1/8"
x 1-5/8". $150.00.

Texide, back.

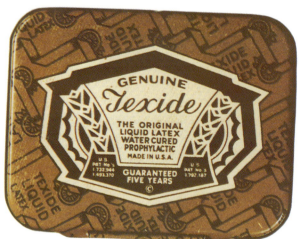

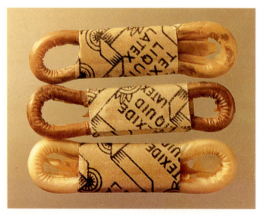

Texide, (paper & rubber) product.

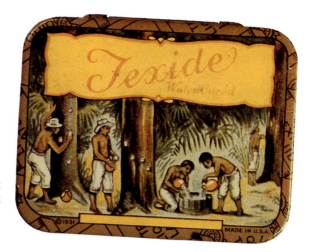

Texide, no guarantee, front. L.E. Shunk Latex Products, Inc. 2-1/8" x 1-5/8". $150.00.

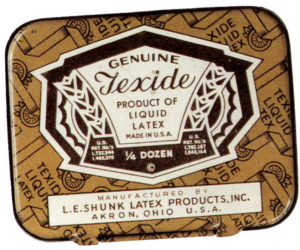

Texide, back.

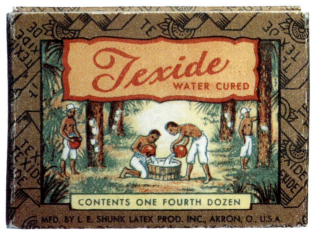

Texide, (paper). L.E. Shunk Latex Products, Inc. 2-1/8" x 1-5/8". $25.00.

TEXIDE

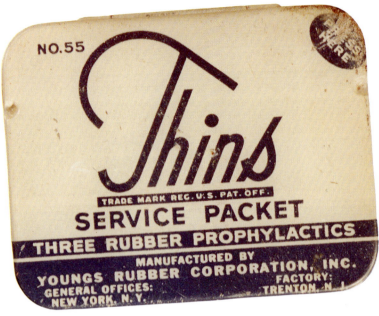

Thins (# 41),
No. 55, front.
Youngs
Rubber
Corporation,
Inc. 2-1/8" x
1-5/8". Rare.

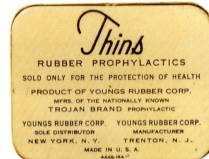

Thins, back.

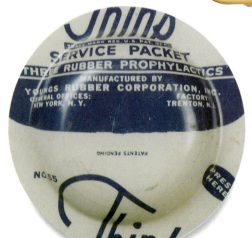

Thins. Service packet
tin. 2" round. Rare.

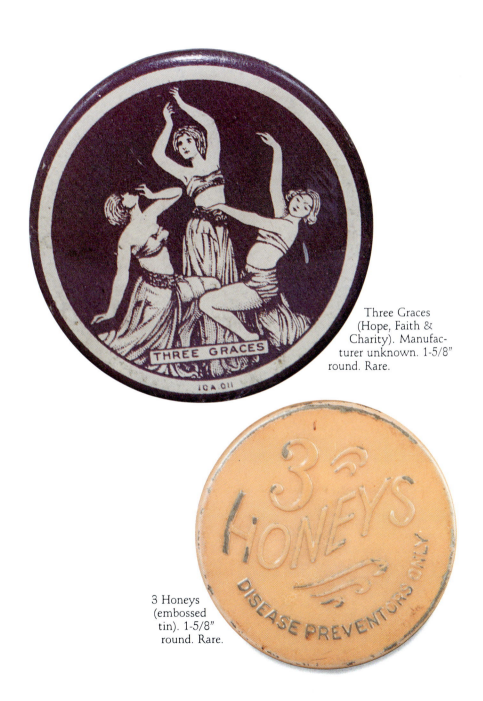

Three Graces
(Hope, Faith &
Charity). Manufac-
turer unknown. 1-5/8"
round. Rare.

3 Honeys
(embossed
tin). 1-5/8"
round. Rare.

THREE HONEYS

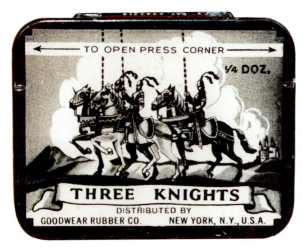

Three Knights (# 41), front. Goodwear Rubber Company. 2-1/8" x 1-5/8". $150.00. U.S. Copyright 371,561. This tin came in two color variations, a white background and a cream background.

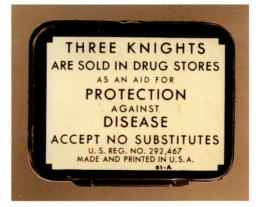

Three Knights, back.

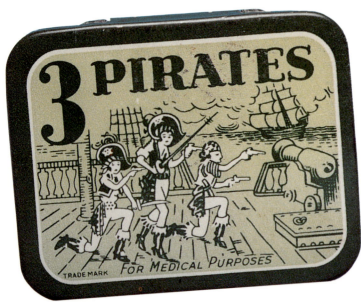

3 Pirates. Akron Rubber Supply Company. 2-1/8" x 1-5/8". Rare.

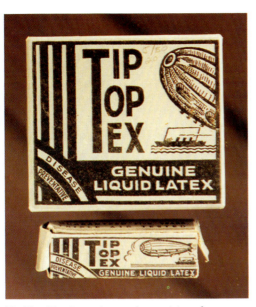

Tip-Top-Tex (paper), one dozen. Manufacturer unknown. Rare. *Courtesy of Richard Oatley.*

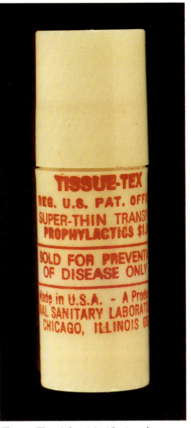

Tissue-Tex (plastic). National Sanitary Labs. 2-1/8" x 1-5/8". $20.00.

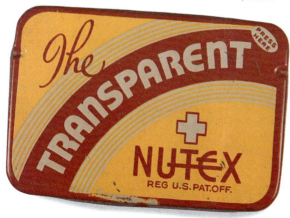

The Transparent Nutex. Nutex Sales Company. 2-5/8" x 1-3/4". $185.00.

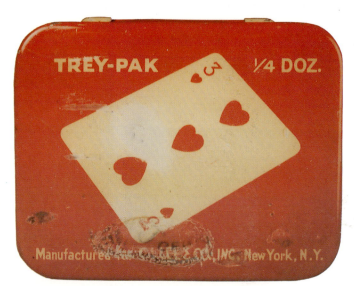

Trey-Pak. C.I. Lee Company, Inc. 2-1/8" x 1-5/8". Rare.

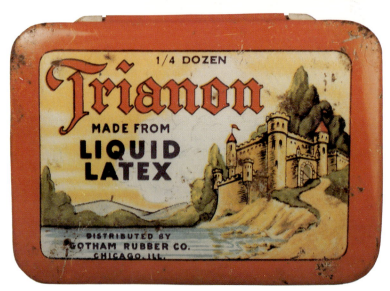

Trianon. Gotham Rubber Company. 2-5/8" x 1-3/4". Rare. The "Magic Kingdom" condom.

Trilby (paper), one dozen envelope. Manufacturer unknown. 2-3/4" x 2-7/16". $15.00. *Courtesy of Richard Oatley.*

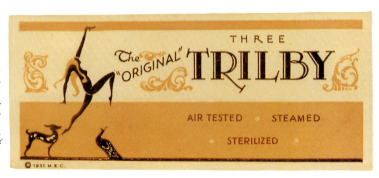

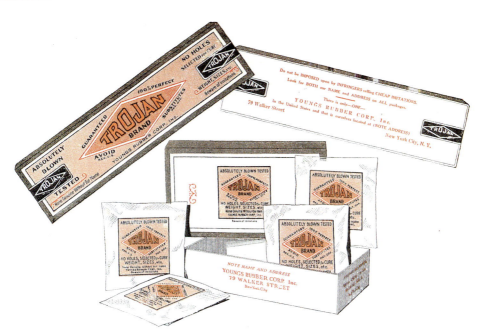

Trojan Brand

Prophylactic Rubber Protectors—Guaranteed 100% Perfect

Finest Quality Obtainable.

Absolutely Blown-tested, Chemically Cured and Scientifically Treated to Neutralize Curing Acids and Prolong the Life of the Goods.

Sold Only to Legitimate Drug Trade

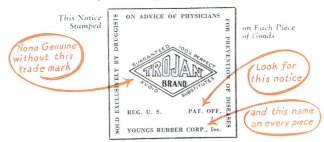

List Prices:

TROJAN BRAND—100%
    Packed Flat (not rolled) in flat box, 1 dozen in box ...... $6.00 per gross

TROJAN BRAND—100%
    Rolled; each piece in individual transparent envelope; 3 envelopes in larger transparent envelope; total of 1 dozen pieces packed in box .... $6.75 per gross

Trojan ad, 1930.

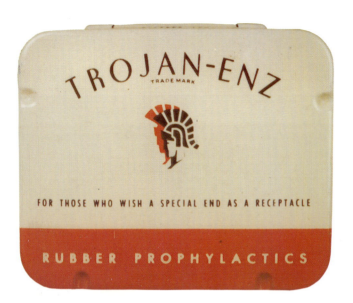

Trojan-Enz. Youngs Rubber Corporation. 2-1/4" x 1-3/4". $150.00. It has been reported that Merle Young made the latex rubber boom of 1930 possible with his testament before Congress that would allow unrestricted sales as long as the container stated "sold for the prevention of disease" with no reference to contraception. However we can find no mention in the Congressional Record for Mr. Young, latex or rubber.

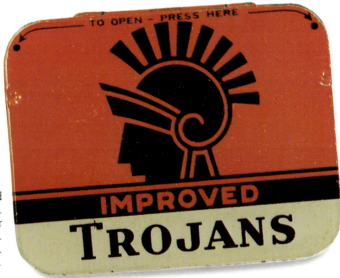

Trojans, Improved (# 41) No. 20. Youngs Rubber Corporation, Inc. 2-1/8" x 1-5/8". $100.00.

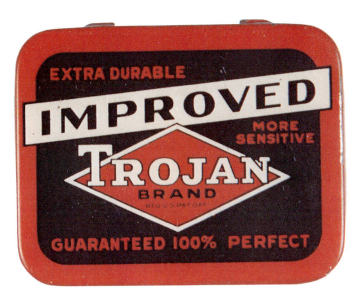

Trojan, Improved,
with diamond,
front. Youngs
Rubber Corporation,
Inc. 2-1/8" x 1-5/8".
$850.00. *Courtesy
Greg Lehne.*

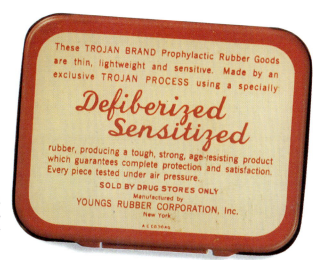

Trojan,
Improved,
back.

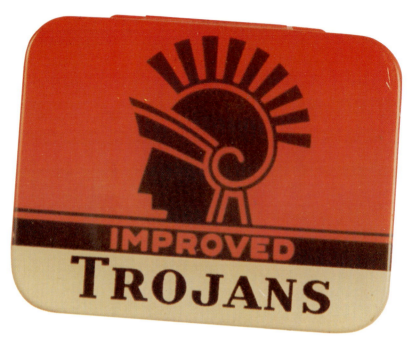

Trojans, Improved, No. 20, front. Youngs Rubber Corporation, Inc. 2-1/8" x 1-5/8". $100.00.

Trojans, Improved (paper), front. Youngs Rubber Corporation, Inc. 2-1/16" x 1-5/8". $25.00.

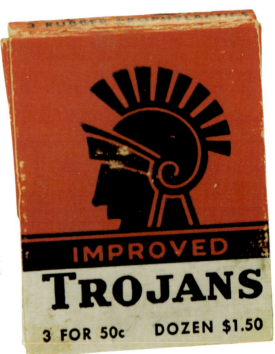

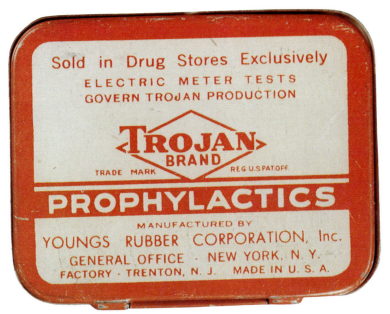

Trojans, Improved,
No. 20, back.

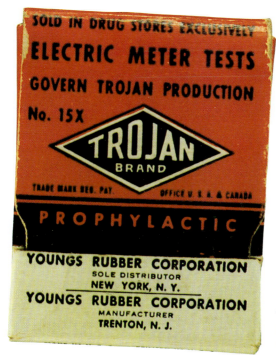

Trojans,
Improved
(paper), back.

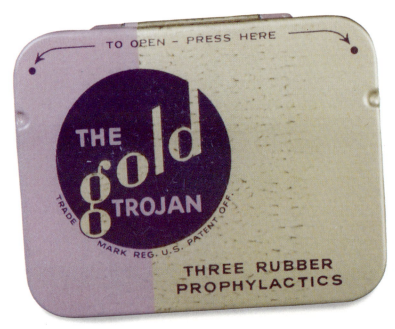

The Gold Trojans
(# 41), violet,
No. 35, front.
Youngs Rubber
Corporation, Inc.
2-1/8" x 1-5/8".
$165.00.

The Gold
Trojans (# 41),
violet, back.

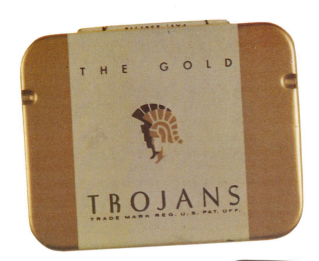

The Gold Trojans (# 41), No. 35, front. Youngs Rubber Corporation, Inc. 2-1/8" x 1-5/8". $75.00.

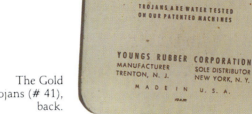

The Gold Trojans (# 41), back.

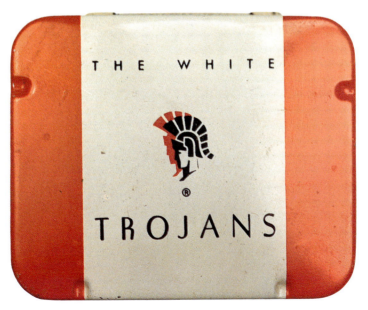

The White Trojans (# 41). Youngs Rubber Corporation, Inc. 2-1/4" x 1-3/4". $100.00.

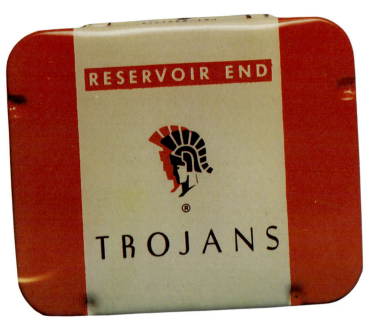

Trojans, Reservoir End. Youngs Rubber
Corporation, Inc. 2-1/4" x 1-3/4". Rare.

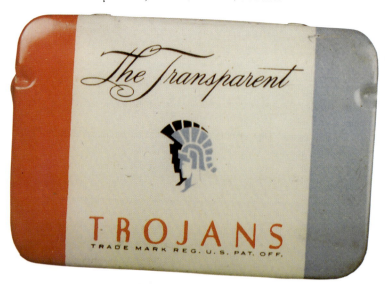

The Transparent Trojans (# 41), No. 40. Youngs
Rubber Corporation, Inc. 2-5/8" x 1-3/4". $200.00.

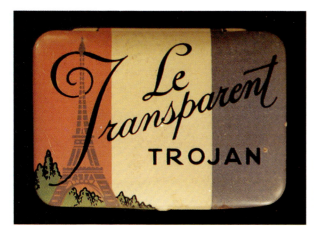

Le Transparent Trojan, front. Youngs Rubber Corporation, Inc. 2-5/8" x 1-3/4". $175.00.

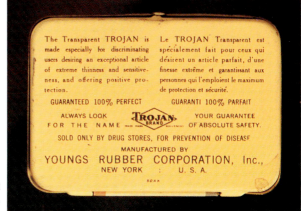

The Transparent TROJAN is made especially for discriminating users desiring an exceptional article of extreme thinness and sensitiveness, and offering positive protection.

Le TROJAN Transparent est spécialement fait pour ceux qui désirent un article parfait, d'une finesse extrême et garantissant aux personnes qui l'emploient le maximum de protection et sécurité.

GUARANTEED 100% PERFECT   GUARANTI 100% PARFAIT

ALWAYS LOOK   **TROJAN**   YOUR GUARANTEE
FOR THE NAME   BRAND   OF ABSOLUTE SAFETY.

SOLD ONLY BY DRUG STORES, FOR PREVENTION OF DISEASE

MANUFACTURED BY

YOUNGS RUBBER CORPORATION, Inc.,
NEW YORK : U.S.A.

Le Transparent Trojan, back.

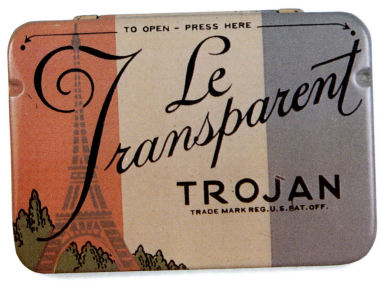

Le Transparent Trojan (# 41). Youngs Rubber Corporation, Inc. 2-5/8" x 1-7/8". $175.00.

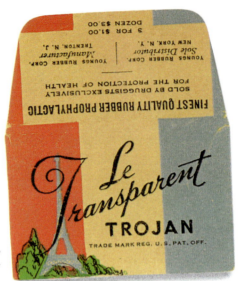

L e Transparent Trojan,
paper envelope.

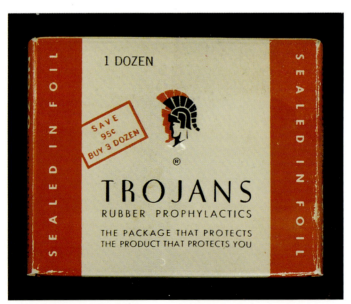

Trojans (paper), 1 Dozen, No. 70. Youngs Rubber
Corporation, Inc. 2-7/8" x 2-3/8". $20.00.

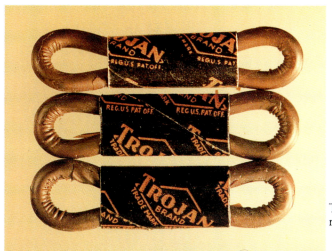

Trojan, (paper & rubber) product.

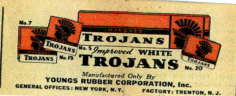

Trojans ad insert, front.

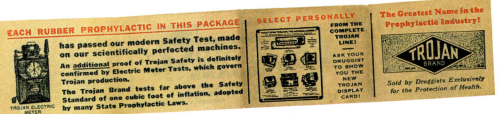

Trojans ad insert, back.

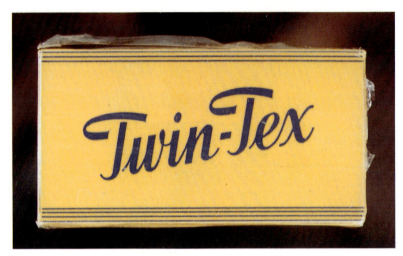

Twin-Tex (paper). Twintex Vendor Manufacturing
Company 2-1/8" x 1-1/16". $5.00.

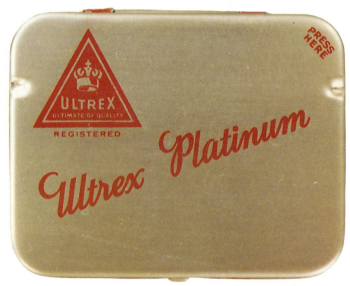

Ultrex Platinum
(# 41), front. Dean
Rubber Manufactur-
ing Company. 2-1/8"
x 1-5/8". $1.00

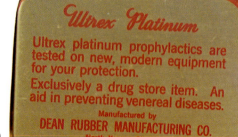

Ultrex Platinum
(# 41), back.

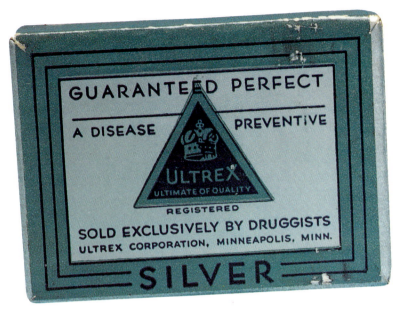

Ultrex Silver (paper). Ultrex Corporation.
2-1/4" x 1-5/8". $35.00.

Ultrex Silver
insert ad.

THE BRAND "ULTREX" IS YOUR GUARANTEE OF THE HIGHEST QUALITY

Every one is air blown tested and free from imperfections. The special Vulco process of manufacturing makes Ultrex the softest, strongest and most sensitive prophylactic on the market. It is odorless and NON-IRRI-TATING because it is rubber in its purest form, and contains the least chemicalization.

YOUR CHOICE

Ultrex comes in three finishes and weights:
Ultrex Silver—white finish—standard weight
Ultrex Gold—Translucent—Somewhat thinner
Ultrex Platinum—Transparent—very thin and Super-sensitive.

For Lubrication use Ultrex Specially prepared lubricating jelly. DO NOT USE VASE-LINE OR OTHER OILY LUBRICANTS as they are harmful to rubber.

VAGINAL ANTISEPTIC

Ultrene Jelly is a highly efficient vaginal antiseptic. It is widely used and recommended by Physicians. Large 4 ounce tube with unbreakable transparent nozzle $1.50 complete. Ask your Druggist.

THE ULTREX CORPORATION
MINNEAPOLIS, MINN.

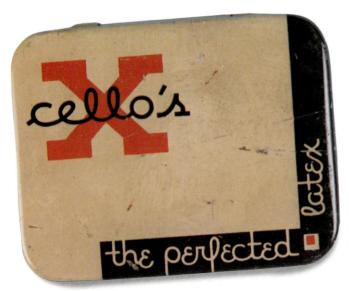

X-Cello's. Killian
Manufacturing
Company. 2-1/8"
x 1-5/8". $250.00.

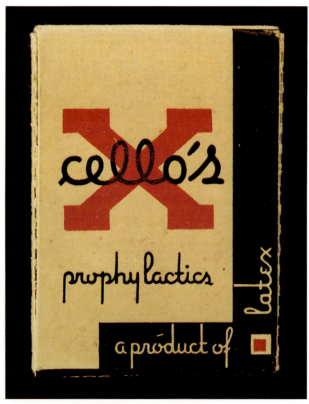

X-Cello's (paper). Killian Manufacturing
Company. 2-1/16" x 1-5/8". $5.00.

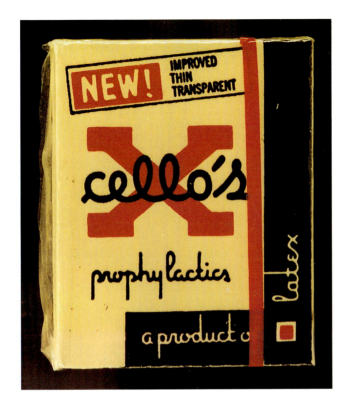

X-Cello's, New (paper). Killian Manufacturing Company. 2-1/16" x 1-5/8". $5.00.

Nur fur die deutsche Wehrmacht bestimmt. Nach Gebrauch sofort zu vernichten. (For The Use of the German War-Machine Exclusively. Dispose of Properly After Use.) Manufacturer unknown. World War II Germany. We close this chapter with a rare German World War II packet that holds two rubbers. Possession by civilians was verboten.

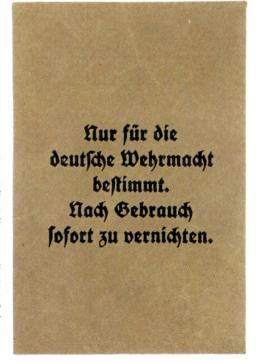

CHAPTER 4
ALUMINUM CONTAINERS

No aluminum tin has been found with a manufacturer's mark. Schmid claimed that they owned "Three Merry Widows." All tins shown are round 1-5/8", friction fit. These cans have either a flat back or concentric rings.

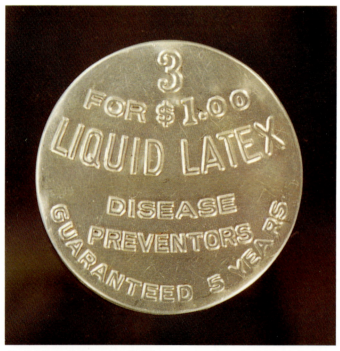

Liquid Latex, Guaranteed 5 Years.
Courtesy of Richard Oatley. $25.00.

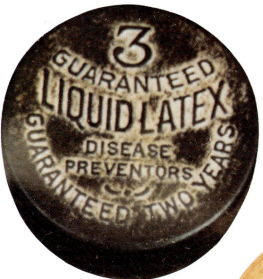

Liquid Latex, Guaranteed 2 Years. $25.00. *Courtesy of Richard Oatley*.

Liquid Latex Prophylactics, Guaranteed 5 Yrs. *Courtesy of Richard Oatley*. $25.00.

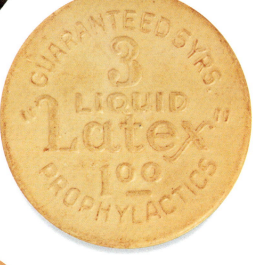

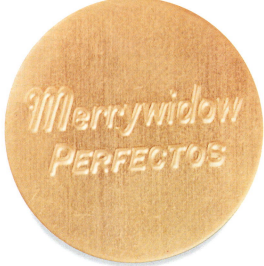

Merry Widows Perfectos. *Courtesy of Richard Oatley*. $30.00.

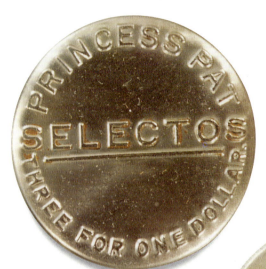

Princess Pat
Selectos. $35.00.

The Real Thing.
$50.00.

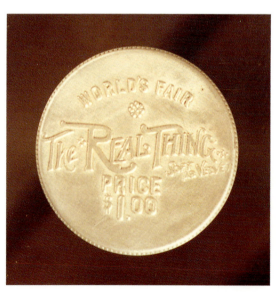

The Real Thing, World's
Fair. *Courtesy of Richard
Oatley.* $25.00.

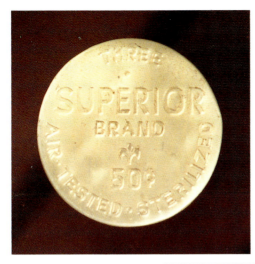

Superior Brand. *Courtesy of Richard Oatley.* $30.00

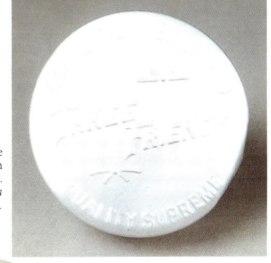

Three Friends. Rare. The slogan: "A true pal when in need" makes this unique. *Courtesy of Steve and Donna Howard.*

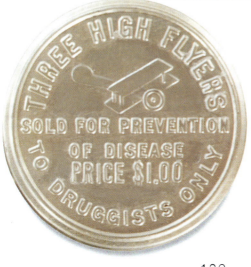

Three High Flyers. $165.00

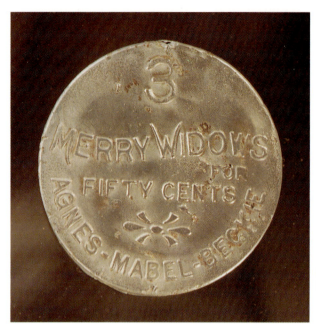

Merry Widows, Agnes-Mable-Beckie. $20.00.

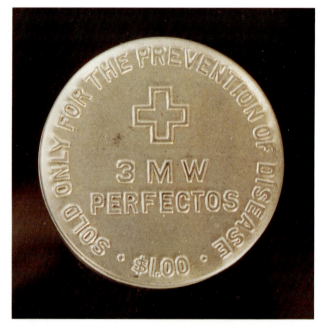

3 M W Perfectos.
$30.00.

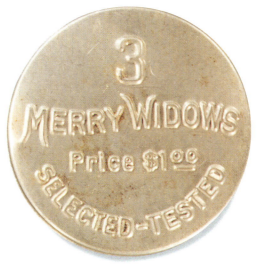

3 Merry Widows,
Selected-Tested.
$25.00.

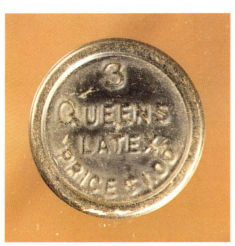

3 Queen's Latex. *Courtesy
of Richard Oatley*. $30.00.

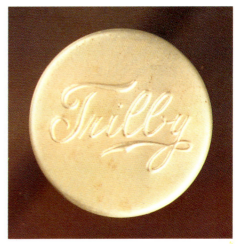

Trilby. *Courtesy of
Richard Oatley*. $30.00

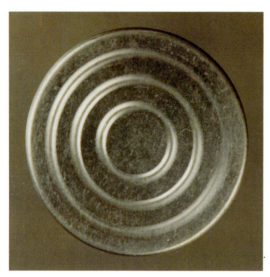

Back with
concentric rings.

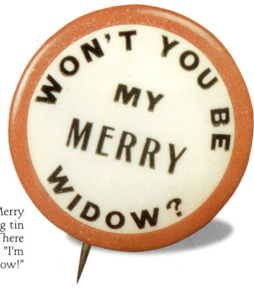

"Won't you be my Merry
Widow?" advertising tin
pinback. 1/4" round. Rare. There
is also a pinback that says "I'm
looking for the Merry Widow!"

142

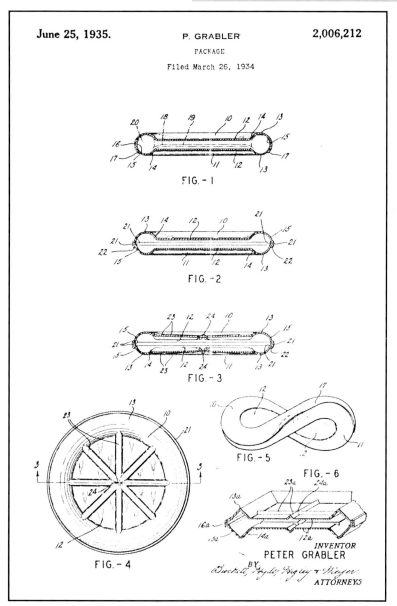

June 25, 1935.

P. GRABLER

2,006,212

PACKAGE

Filed March 26, 1934

FIG. - 1

FIG. - 2

FIG. - 3

FIG. - 4

FIG. - 5

FIG. - 6

INVENTOR
PETER GRABLER
BY
ATTORNEYS

Illustration from U.S. patent 2,006,212.

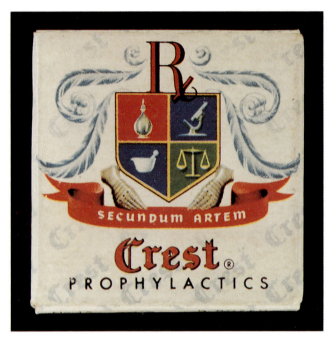

Crest, front. National Hygienic Products
Corporation. 1-3/4" x 1-3/4". $20.00

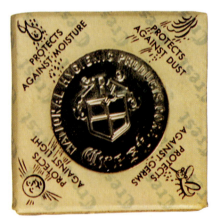

Crest, back.

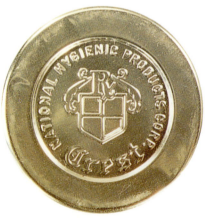

Crest contents.
1-5/8" x 1-5/8".

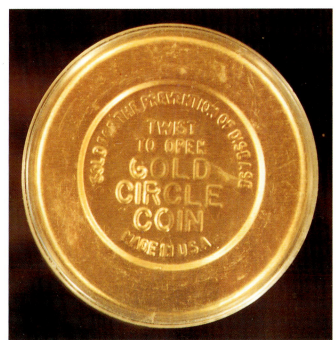

Gold Circle Coin.
Circle Rubber
Corporation.
$30.00.

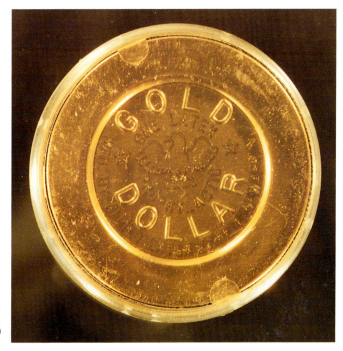

Gold Dollar.
Allied Latex.
$10.00

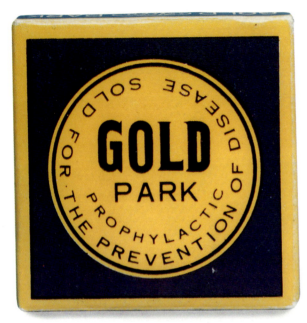

Gold Park (paper box).
Manufacturer unknown.
1-3/4" x 1-3/4". $20.00.

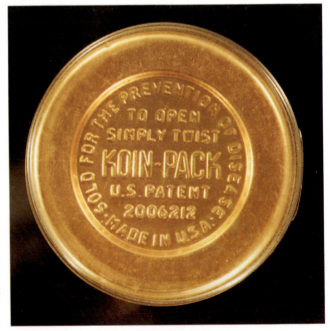

Koin-Pack. L.E.
Shunk Latex
Products, Inc. 1-5/8"
round. $15.00.

CHAPTER 6

CHEMICAL PROPHYLACTICS

Kept alive by the army, chemical prophylactics were used principally to ward off venereal disease after sexual contact...kind of like closing the barn doors after the horses have fled. Two major brands were used, Dough Boy and Hy-Gee. Some say that Hy-Gee is the note you hit when you applied it. The instructions warn of a slight burning...but suggest that it is better than the alternative.

Dough-Boy Prophylactic (paper). The Reese Chemical Company. 3-5/8" x 2-5/16". $40.00. Dough-Boy comes with a cloth bag & draw string to complete the job.

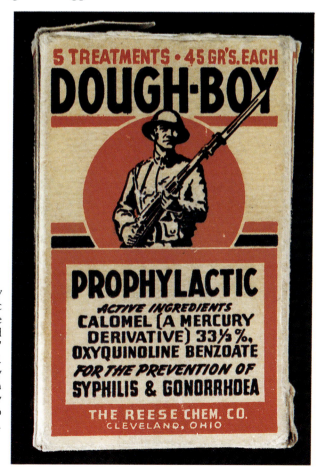

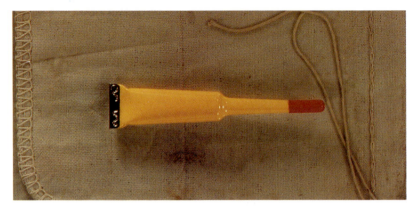

Dough-Boy Prophylactic (paper)
pouch. 3-5/8" x 1-3/8". $10.00.

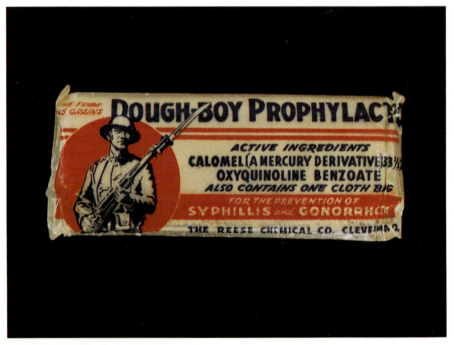

Dough-Boy Prophylactic (metal,
plastic & cotton) tube & bag.

Opposite:
Dough-Boy Prophylactic.
Instructions.

DOUGHBOY PROPHYLACTIC

DIRECTIONS

1. Urinate. 2. Wash external parts thoroughly with soap and water, lathering well for several minutes; then dry well.

3. Squeeze a small amount of the ointment from the tube and lubricate the tip of the tube so that it slips into the canal easily. Next squeeze about ⅓ of the contents of the tube into the canal, then close the lips of the canal with the thumb and forefinger to prevent the ointment from escaping, and massage well so as to spread the ointment thoroughly over the walls and into the spongy tissues of the canal.

4. Squeeze the remainder of the ointment on the outside, covering all parts and rub in well, especially where germs might locate.

5. Attach bag for cleanliness and allow it to remain for several hours.

NOTICE: When Doughboy Prophylactic is squeezed into the canal a slight "burning" is felt, for a few seconds only. Such irritation of the tender tissues is certain to follow the use of an effective preparation, so do not allow a few seconds of discomfort to alarm or influence you.

Use immediately if possible, if not, be sure to use within an hour after exposure. However, if you should fail or neglect to use within an hour, use as soon as you can for it still may be possible to secure protection if not delayed too long.

MODE D'EMPLOI

Un tube de "Dough-Boy" Prophylactique
Agents actifs—Calomel (Protochlorure de mercure)
33⅓ % — oxyquinoline de benzoate
Pour la prevention de la Syphillis et de la Blennorragie

1. Urinez. 2. Lavez bien avec du savon et de l'eau froide; si possible savonnez pendant plusieurs minutes; puis séchez soigneusement. 3. Sortez une petite quantité de l'onguent du tube, et enduisez en l'extrémité de façon à ce qu'il glisse facilement dans le canal. Ensuite videz ⅓ environ du contenu du tube dans le canal, puis fermez les levres avec les doigts pour empêcher la pommade d'en sortir, massez soigneusement pour faire pènètrer celle-ci dans les parois et le tissus poreux du canal. 4. Videz le restant de la pommade sur les parties extèrieures, en en recouvrant toutes les parties et en frottant bien soigneusement, spécialement où les germes peuvent être localisés. 5. Attachez le sac et laissez le ainsi pendant plusieurs heures.

A employer immediatement après avoir été exposè, sinon soyez sur de l'employer une heure après.

DIREZIONE

Un tubo 45 Grani Proglattico "Dugh-Boy"
Ingredient Attivi—Calomel (un derivato di mescurio) 33⅓ % —Benzoato exiquinilino
Per la prevenzione della Sifilide e della Gonorrea

1. Orinate. 2. Lavate la parte con sapone ed acqua calda; se possibile insaponate bene per diversi minuti; poscia asciugate per bene. 3. Spremete una piccola quantita' dell'unguento dal tubo e ungete la punta del tubo stesso, in modo che entri facilmente nel canale. Indi spremete circa un terzo del contenuto del tubo dentro il canale, e quindi chiudete la punta del canale con le dita, per impedire che l'unguento esca; massaggiate bene per far penetrare l'unguento in ogni parte, compreso il tessuto spugnoso del canale. 4. Spremete il rimanente dell'unguento sopra le parti esterne, coprendole e massaggiandole per bene, specialmente dove i germi si possano annidare. 5. Applicate la borsa per non sporcarvi e tenetevela per alcune ore.

Usatelo immediatamente, se vi e' possibile; caso contrario fate in modo di usarlo entro un'ora dopo il contatto.

DIRECCIONES

Un tubo 45 granos Profiláctico "Dough-Boy"
Ingredientes activos—Calomel (Derivativo mercúrico) 33⅓ %—Benvoato oxiquinolino
Para la prevención de Sífilis y Gonorrea

1. Orine. 2. Lávese bien con agua fría y jabón; si es posible, lávese con la espuma del jabón por varios minutos; séquese bien. 3. Saque un poco del ungüento apretando el tubo y lubrique la punta de éste, para que pueda entrar fácilmente en el canal. Apriete hasta meter una tercera parte del contenido del tubo en el canal, cierre bien apretando con el pulgar y el dedo índice para evitar que el ungüento se salga y masaje bien para que el ungüento se esparza por todas las paredes y membranas suaves del canal. 4. Saque el resto del ungüento y espárzalo por toda la parte exterior, cubiendo bien todas las partes que se hayan expuesto y masaje hasta estar seguro que estas están bien cubiertas. 5. Aplíquese la bolsa o saco para protección y déjelo puesto por varias horas.

Use este ungüento inmediatamente si es posible, pero si no, esté seguro de usarlo dentro de una hora después de ser expuesto.

GEBRAUCHSANWEISUNG

Eine roehre 45 Grane "Dough-Boy"
Vorbeugungsmittel—Wirksame bestandteile—Calomel (ein Quecksilberderivate) 33⅓ %—Oxychinolines Benzoesalz
Zur verhütung von Syphillis and Gonorrhoe

1. Urinieren. 2. Gruendlich waschen mit Seife und kaltem Wasser; womoeglich gut schaeumen einige Minuten; dann sorgsam trocknen. 3. Ein wenig von der Salbe aus der Roehre ausdruecken, um die Spitze der Roehre geschmeidig zu machen, damit sie leicht in den Gang hineinrutschen kann. Zunaechst 1/3 von dem Inhalt der Roehre in den Gang ausdruecken dann die Lippen des Ganges mit den Daumen und dem Zeigefinger zusperren, um das Ausrennen der Salbe zu verhindern; und gut massieren, bis die Salbe gruendlich ueber die Waende und in die schwammartigen Geweben des Ganges verbreitet wird. 4. Das uebrige der Salbe auf der Aussenseite pressen, alle Teile damit zudecken, und gut einreiben, besonders wo Bakterien sich ansieden koennten. 5. Einen Sack anbinden der Reinlichkeit wegen, und ihn lassen einige Stunden.

Womoeglich sofort gebrauchen; wenn nicht, innerhalb einer Stunde nach dem Ausgesetzsein verwenden.

Manufactured by THE REESE CHEMICAL CO., Cleveland, O.

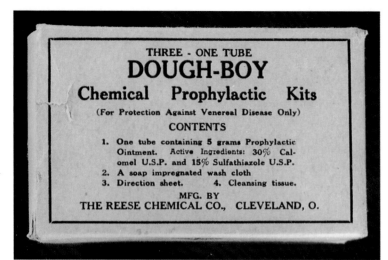

THREE - ONE TUBE
DOUGH-BOY
Chemical Prophylactic Kits
(For Protection Against Venereal Disease Only)
CONTENTS
1. One tube containing 5 grams Prophylactic Ointment. Active Ingredients: 30% Calomel U.S.P. and 15% Sulfathiazole U.S.P.
2. A soap impregnated wash cloth
3. Direction sheet.   4. Cleansing tissue.

MFG. BY
THE REESE CHEMICAL CO.,   CLEVELAND, O.

Dough-Boy Chemical Prophylactic Kits, number 1715 (paper), front. Reese Chemical Company. $10.00.

Dough-Boy Chemical Prophylactic Kits, number 1715 (paper), back.

THE PROPHYLACTIC OINTMENT CONTAINED IN THIS KIT CONFORMS WITH ARMY PRO-KIT SPECIFICATIONS.

No. 1715 - 29 JUNE 1944

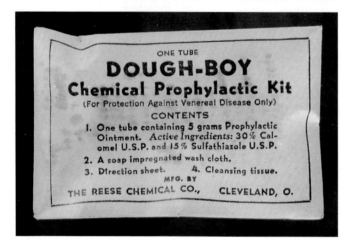

ONE TUBE
DOUGH-BOY
Chemical Prophylactic Kit
(For Protection Against Venereal Disease Only)
CONTENTS
1. One tube containing 5 grams Prophylactic Ointment. Active Ingredients: 30% Calomel U.S.P. and 15% Sulfathiazole U.S.P.
2. A soap impregnated wash cloth.
3. Direction sheet.   4. Cleansing tissue.

MFG. BY
THE REESE CHEMICAL CO.,   CLEVELAND, O.

Dough-Boy Chemical Prophylactic Kits, number 1715 (paper), packet.

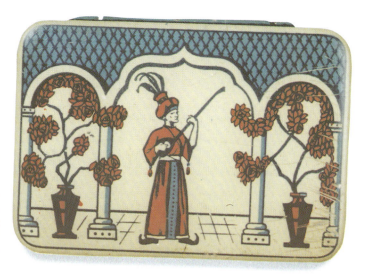

Hy-Gee. The Hygee Company. 2-5/8" x 1-3/4". $100.00. Hy-Gee came in another size, 2-3/4" x 1-3/4" and 2-1/8" x 1-5/8".

Hy-Gee. Instructions, front in English, back in Spanish.

HY-GEE

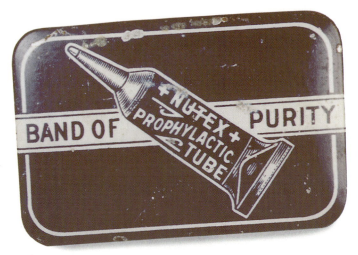

Nutex Prophylactic Tube, inside "Band of Purity" tin. Nutex Sales Company. 2-3/4" x 1-3/4". $250.00.

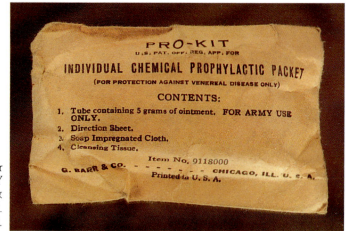

Pro-Kit. Item number 9118000. FOR ARMY USE ONLY. G. Barr & Company. 3-1/2" x 2". $10.00.

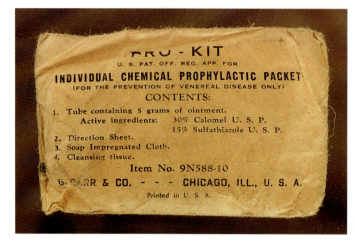

Pro-Kit. Item number 9N588-10. G. Barr & Company. 3-1/2" x 2". $10.00.

CHAPTER 7

KIND OF, BUT NOT QUITE

Now that we've let rubbers out of the closet, these guys were also found gasping for air... not really rubbers, but rubber related.

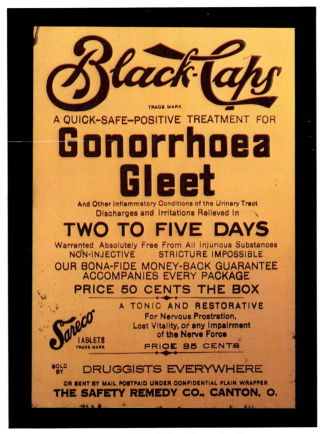

Black-Caps (metal) Sign. The Safety Remedy Company. 9-1/2" x 7. If you forgot your rubbers you could turn to "Black Caps" or "Okay Specific". The match box holder for Pabst's has a Calendar for 1929 & 1930 on the back.

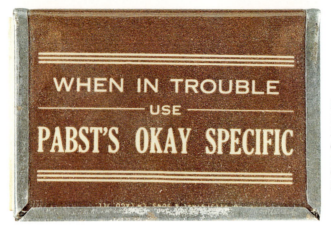

Pabst's Okay Specific (metal, plastic & paper), Match box holder, calendar for 1929 & 1930 on back. Pabst's Chemical Company 2-3/8" x 1-5/8". $20.00.

Right:
Sanitary Health Sponge. Manufacturer unknown. 1-3/4" round. $80.00. This tin still holds a pink net bag with a long string. You could spend three to five years in a federal prison for including instructions with this contraceptive device.

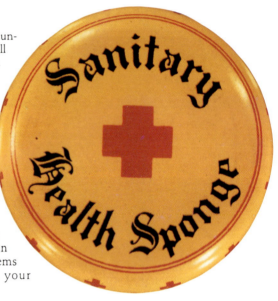

Below:
Ergoapiol. Martin H. Smith Company. 3-3/4" x 2". $20.00. Ergapiol says this stuff is for amenorrhea? Let's see here in my dictionary... "Amenorrhea: Abnormal absence of the menstrual discharge." Ye Gods Martha! This is an abortion drug! This stuff is made from Ergot (a fungus of rye) from which L.S.D. can be extracted. Usually these kinds of items were sold as "female pills". Ask your druggist...he knows.

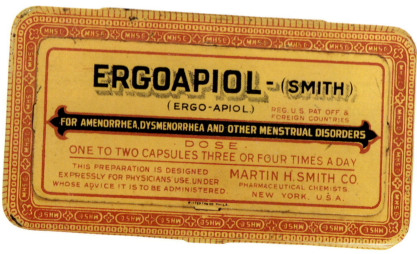

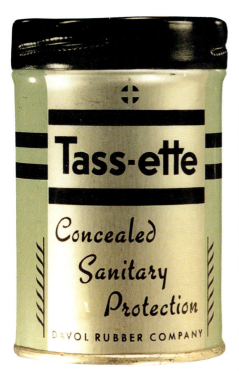

Tass-ette. Davol Rubber Company.
3" x 2-1/8" round. $30.00. Tass-ette
patented in 1936. Invented by a ballerina
and her brother, a gynecologist.

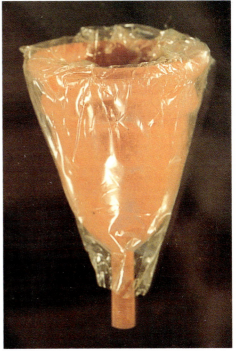

Tass-ette product.

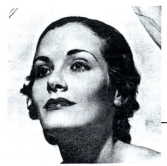

A SHADOW DISAPPEARS

Tass-ette instructions.

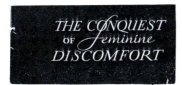

THE CONQUEST
OF *feminine*
DISCOMFORT

The *Tass-ette is made in one
size only from high-grade rubber, the quality of which is
fully guaranteed. It will last a
year or more, and thus effects
a material saving in the cost
of menstrual protection. The
Tass-ette is on sale at better
drug stores and department
stores; No. 365, price $1.00.
* Patent Pending.

Moisten the Tass-ette and press its sides together, as in the first picture. With sides pressed
flat, fold them over again, as in the second picture. Hold cup as shown in third picture, and
while in a stooping, relaxed position, insert
slowly into the vagina. Press gently upward as
far as fingers will permit, then release the sides
of the Tass-ette until the cup is completely open.

Now push gently upward on tip, with a side-
to-side motion, until the cup is a little beyond
the comfortable height. Draw tip slightly forward until cup is securely seated in the walls
of the vagina just below the cervix (mouth of
the uterus). The tip is then within easy reach
for removal. The Tass-ette must be in an upright position, forming a sealed receptacle. No
part of it is exposed when correctly seated.
Observe illustration showing cup in proper
position.

Remember that it is not necessary to remove
the Tass-ette for normal elimination of the colon
or urinary canal.

To remove the cup, draw the tip gently and
slowly toward the back, in the direction of the
rectum. This tilts the rim of the cup and releases
the vacuum. Now pull gently downward from

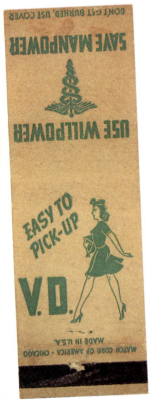

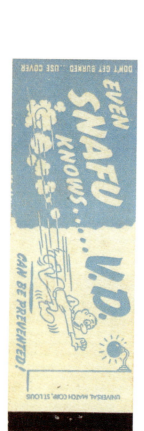

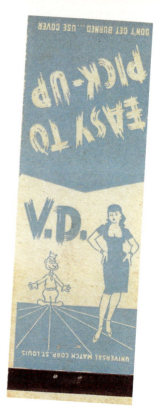

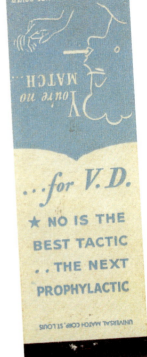

Four World War II match book covers, little reminders from the "American War Machine." Go ask your dad what SNAFU means.

RUBBER MANUFACTURERS AND DISTRIBUTORS

Frank Aaronoff, New York, New York
    Kamels.
Akron Rubber Supply Company, Chicago, Illinois
    Akron Tourist Tubes
    3 Pirates
Allied Latex Corporation, East Newark and Haskell, New Jersey
    Gold Dollar
    Red Bird
    Seal-Tite
Allied Latex Sales, New York, New York
    Royal Knight (Knight)
    Clear-Tone
Allied Latex Sales Division, New York, New York
    Gems
    Smithies
American Hygienic Company, Baltimore, Maryland
    De-Luxe Blue-Ribbon
Aronab Products Company, San Francisco
    Romeos
Arrow Rubber Corporation, New York, New York
    Nunbetter
Barr, G. & Company, Chicago, Illinois
    Pro-Kit

H.L. Blake, Hot Springs, Arkansas
    Big Chief
    B.C.
Central Sundries Inc., New York, New York
    Royal Knight (castle)
Chandler Distributors, Saint Louis, Missouri
    Par-X
Circle Rubber Corporation, Newark, New Jersey
    Essex
    Gold Circle Coin
    Prince
    Red Circle
    Stubs
Crown Rubber Company, Akron, Ohio
    Esquire
    Gold-Pak
Dean Rubber Manufacturing Company, North Kansas City, Missouri
    Parisians
    Peacock
    Rainbow
    Sekurity
    Ultrex Platinum
Department Sales Company, New York, New York
    Duble-Tip

Excello Hygienic Products Corp., New York, New York
Sovereigns

Feather-Tex Rubber Company, New York, New York
Feather-Tex

Foster Rubber Company, Boston, Massachusetts
Foster Rubber

Gold-Tex Rubber Company, New York, New York
Gold-Tex

Goodwear Rubber Company, Inc., New York, New York
Chariots
Stags
Three Graces
3 Knights

Gotham Sales Company, Inc., New York, New York
Tally-Ho

Gotham Rubber Company, Chicago, Illinois & New York, New York
Saf-T-Way
Trianon

Hygee Company, The. Kansas City, Missouri
Hy-Gee

International Distributors, Memphis, Tennessee
Rough Rider

Julius Schmid, Inc., New York, New York
Cadets
Ramses
Sheik
Sphinx
Sphinx, 3
XXXX (4X)

Killian Manufacturing Company, Akron Ohio
Apris
Derbies
Napoleons
Romeos
Silver-Tex
Silver-Tex De-Luxe
X-Cello's

C.L. Lee & Company, New York, New York
Trey-Pak

M & M Rubber Company, Kansas City, Missouri
Spartans
Tomahawk

Lorica Laboratories Inc., Jersey City, New Jersey
"Shorts"

158

L.J. McFadden Company, Cedar Rapids, Iowa
    Silver Knight
Mayfair Chemical Corporation, New York, New York
    Silver-Town
Midwest Drug Company, Minneapolis, Minnesota
    Aristocrat
Modern Distributing Company, Detroit, Michigan
    Modern-Tex
National Hygienic Products Corporation,
    Champ (baseball, boxing, football, golf)
    Crest (koin)
National Sanitary Laboratories, Inc., Chicago, Illinois
    Tissue-Tex
National Sanitary Sales Inc., Chicago, Illinois
    Protex
    Spares
Nutex Sales Company, Philadelphia, Pennsylvania
    Drug-Pak
    Lifeguards
    Nu-Tips
    Prophylactic Tube, Brand of

Purity
    Radium, The
    Transparent, The
Olympic Vending Company, Kansas City, Missouri
    Olympic
Peerless Products Company, Kansas City, Missouri
    Certex
Prophylactic Company Inc., New York, New York
    Pro-Fo
W.H. Reed & Company Inc., Atlanta Georgia
    Golden Pheasant
    Pan
    Surette
Reese Chemical Company, Cleveland, Ohio
    Dough-Boy
Robert J. Pierce Inc., New York, New York
    Hercules
    Optimus
Schaeffer Products, Cleveland, Ohio
    Blue Goose
    Gensco

BIBLIOGRAPHY

Bergevin, Al. *Drugstore Tins and their Prices*. Radnor, Pennsylvania: Wallace-Homestead, 1990.

Burke, James Lee. *Connections*. Boston: Little, Brown and Company 1978.

Dodge, Fred. *Antiques Tins*. Paducah, Kentucky: Collector Books, 1995

Haefs, Gadriele. *Dein Kondom-das unbekannte Wesen*. Germany: Buntbuch Verlag, 1985. English Translation, *Johnny Come Lately: A Short History of the Condom*. London, England: The Journeyman Press Ltd, 1987.

Secrest, Clark, AKA Nosmo King. *Tintype*.

Verdi, Giuseppe. "La Donna e Moblie" from *Rigoletto*. Sung by Luciano Pavarotti.

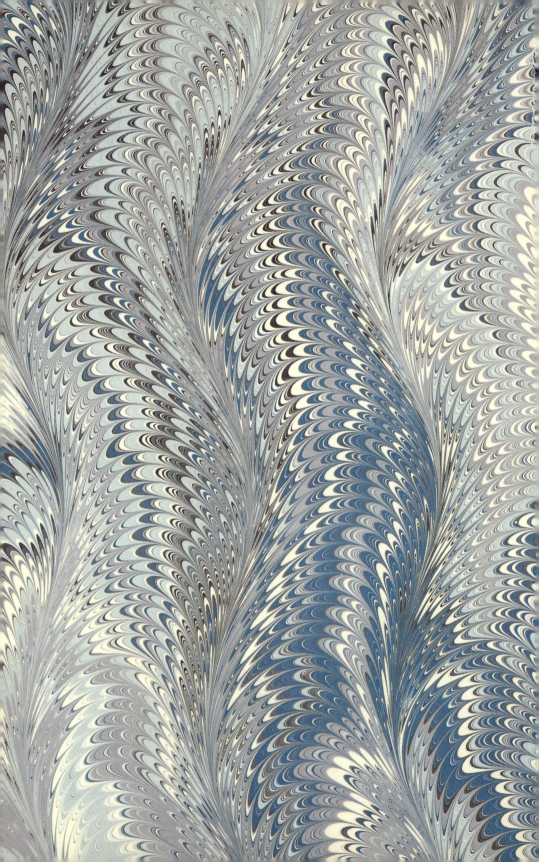